Journey to Fitness

Chronicles of a Working Woman

Linda S. Jassmond Lanfear

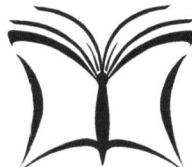

alexemi
PUBLISHING
Exton, Pennsylvania

First Edition

Library of Congress Control Number

LCCN 2008942602

ISBN 978-0-9815954-2-9

Published by:

Alexemi Publishing
P.O. Box 1266
Exton, PA 19341
www.alexemipublishing.com

Book cover design and interior layout: Ronda Taylor, Taylor by Design

Printed in the U.S.A. 2009

For Suzanne, you are an inspiration.

Contents

May

June

July

Epilogue

Prologue
by Linda S. Jassmond Lanfear

Immediately after taking my first aerobics class in 1984, I went to a fast food restaurant to order a cheeseburger and fries. Showing some restraint and to offset the fries, I opted for a diet soda instead of a milk shake.

Fortunately, I caught the fitness bug back then, learned how to teach aerobics classes and learned how to eat healthfully. Years later, I started a personal training business with the intent of sharing my knowledge with others.

After I had been working as a trainer for a while, the idea came to me to chronicle a client's daily struggle to get in shape. There was no guarantee the client would succeed, so the book could easily be a flop. Then again, even if the client failed, it would be a learning experience for both the reader and for me. It was a chance I was willing to take.

Introducing Suzanne…She is a CPA who works outside the home. She has three boys who are involved in sports and other activities. Suzanne has a husband, a dog, a very social family life and is active in her church, business and community. She loves food and everything about it—she even reads cookbooks for enjoyment. Having tried on numerous occasions, she decided she just didn't have time to exercise.

Turn the page to follow Suzanne on her journey.

Introduction:

Preparing For Her Journey

I had known Suzanne for years and had always admired her as a businesswoman. When I was looking for people to help me with my personal training business, she immediately came to mind.

The September before our fitness journey began, I sent Suzanne an email asking her if she would be interested in coming to work with me. This was her answer:

> "I hope all is well with you. I am getting back into my normal work routine now that the kids are all in school. They are in three different schools this year and I realized how quiet it is in the morning because they don't see each other—one leaves and the next one gets up, etc.

> "I gave your offer about training to be a personal trainer a LOT of thought. What I realized though is that I don't think I would be doing the job for the right reasons. For me, I think it would be more about me, and me getting in shape, and me getting the exercise and me making money and unfortunately less about the person I should be helping. I still think my goal would be to have a personal trainer of my own. That just doesn't sound like the right attitude for the job. I sincerely appreciate your thought (although at first it did seem like quite a stretch for me) and respect. I think I am better suited for the CPA world.

> "Thank you for everything and hopefully I'll see you soon.

> "Best regards,

> Suz"

After receiving her response, I suggested that we start working together in January, with me as her personal trainer. We could see each other once a month and she could share with me the challenges a working mother of three faces. She agreed so I asked her to start journaling right away, even before our first meeting.

Sunday, September 10

Suzanne's Journal Notes …

"My whole body hang-up has to do with my stomach—belly—waistline—whatever you want to call it. The clothes just seem to get tighter and tighter around the waist. The sad part is that I think I know what I need to do, it's just doing it. I eat really well—as in good-for-me foods—but my portion control is a BIG problem."

Monday, October 2

Suzanne's Journal Notes …

"Okay, I'll start today. I promised Linda I would start journaling but I haven't really made the effort yet. I always say I want to journal, but I don't ever do it consistently. I am going to start with the random thoughts that have been going through my head for weeks.

"Some days I feel like I can do it all and other days I wonder how I'll ever get organized and get accomplished what I want to do. Some days my appearance doesn't bother me and other days I still long to have a body like Cindy Crawford. The way I see it for me, the key to weight loss is portion control and organization. If I would just eat less and be prepared with the 'right' kinds of food to eat, I should lose weight.

"I still don't know how to put exercise into a daily routine. And I am nervous because today, I really don't even want to. I was trying to fit in the 20-minute Pilates DVD. I caught

a cold and that seemed to be the end of that. If I can't even commit to 20 minutes, how can I ever expect to improve my shape?

"I also have a tremendous love for food. I love to cook it, eat it and shop for it—all of it. So it is really hard for me to avoid it."

Saturday, November 4

I emailed Suzanne asking how she was doing and got quite a response:

"Truthfully, feeling fat and sluggish and slightly overwhelmed at the moment. I don't know why some days I feel like I can conquer the world and other days I feel completely defeated. I heard a small piece of the Oprah show the other day about dieting. The doctor she was interviewing said that a woman's waistline should be under 32.5 inches. Well, not mine, not even close, it is 36 inches—how embarrassing was that? And now we are headed into the holiday season, which is definitely not good for my waistline. My sister's advice is to stop worrying so much about food and worry more about the exercise. Linda, I am just stuck on when I am going to exercise—faithfully. I can do anything for a short time, but how to maintain??? Thanks for asking!"

Wednesday, December 20

I sent Suzanne an email asking how she was, and told her I was looking forward to working with her in the New Year. Then I got a little nervous because there was no response for days. A few more days went by and I had this sinking feeling that maybe Suzanne was backing out. It was one thing for her to have said 'yes' to me months ago and quite another when the time was approaching. I know her and I knew she could do this, so I hoped she would respond.

Monday, January 1

I sent an email to Suzanne wishing her Happy New Year and asked her to give me a choice of dates for us to get together:

> "Happy New Year to you too!! I apologize for not wishing you a Merry Christmas before the holidays. I hope you had a wonderful holiday. Ours was terrific! Tomorrow the routine starts all over again and I am so ready to get busy with myself. I had outpatient surgery on December 29. Not a big deal and all is well, but I am not supposed to exercise for three weeks. I have to schedule my follow-up appointment, and I will clarify, but I am assuming that I can still take some brisk walks. So my question is; do you want to meet pre or post my three-week restriction time? I do not have scheduled hours at my office on Fridays, so Friday is my best day and I am available on Monday afternoons. I can't wait!!! And, I want to know exactly how I can best help you in your research. I have done lousy in the journal department, but have resolved to figure out when to get that scheduled in my day. Thank you again!"

Suzanne's Journal Notes ...

"11:00 a.m. breakfast: two pieces of French toast with syrup, eight ounces of cranberry-pineapple juice and water. 2:00 p.m. lunch: eight chicken wings with blue cheese dressing, celery, caffeine-free diet cola, four cookies and more water. 7:00 p.m. dinner: two and a half slices of roasted pork, sauerkraut, mashed potatoes, green beans, half-inch slice of ice cream cake and water."

Tuesday, January 2

I sent Suzanne an email confirming that we would meet on Friday, January 5. I asked for pictures of her in bike pants and a sports bra or something revealing with a front view, right profile, back view and left profile. She responded to my email:

> *"Sounds great and sounds yucky (in that order), but I'll do it. See you then."*

She was excited about our meeting, except for the photos, which is common. With this type of attitude, I knew I was getting Suzanne at the right time in her life—the time when she's ready to change for the better.

Thursday, January 4

Suzanne's Journal Notes ...

> *"I was thinking about this today...I think my life is about balance and choices. For example, yesterday I was feeling out of balance with my son Griffin, so I made the choice to go to his away wrestling match and cut my work day a little short. Also part of keeping balance in my life is trying to keep as much order in the house as possible (not very good at it), but again I chose to be a little late to work so that I could stop at the post office, drop off the dry cleaning and go to the store for a new family calendar. At the time, the order at home was more important than getting to work on time, so I made that choice to be late."*

The next day, Suzanne's journey began.

January:
The Journey Begins

Our First Meeting, Friday, January 5

We hugged hello and Suzanne said, "I'm obsessed with food. I was thinking about this today…. I think my life is about balance and choices." Suzanne feels her life is all about the choices she makes and the consequences of her choices. I wish I had a tape recorder because I couldn't write as fast as we were talking. This one-hour meeting turned out to be two hours and it set the stage for an interesting journey.

My first topic was family medical history. Suzanne is 5'7" and her starting weight was 157 pounds. Her weight had been fairly constant for the past few years. Her father passed away of a heart attack at age 61. "Mom's great. She's 69, is very, very disciplined and eats like a saint." With those types of comments, we'd be talking more about her mom and her mom's relationship with food.

I asked about goals. "Hum. It's not really about weight. It's about being comfortable in my skin. I walk heavy and feel heavy. My greatest success would be figuring out how to fit fitness into my schedule on a regular basis and be excited about it. I also want life balance."

Suzanne liked taking classes at a gym because she used the other women to motivate and push her. She likes to walk, swim and hit tennis balls; she loves being outside. "Anything I could do with my kids," was her response when we talked about exercise and her boys, who are 14, 12 and 6. The boys play sports: soccer, basketball, gymnastics, wrestling and more. "I don't like it so forced," she continued about exercise. Suzanne would like to run but has never been able to, even when she was younger. Her family has no formal exercise equipment at home.

Suzanne and her husband want to do ballroom dancing, so I encouraged her to sign up. She was considering joining a fitness club with her 14-year-old because she thought he could motivate her. She talked several times about exercise not being a priority because of everything else going on in her life. This lack of priority is such a common comment from moms; they put themselves last. Suzanne liked the idea of doing only 5-10 minutes of exercise several times throughout the day. Ideally I'd like to have her exercise three to four times a week for an hour, but that just isn't going to happen now. So, we're starting out slow to create a habit.

"Even the dog is lazy." I suggested she engage the dog in her exercise program—throw him a ball or take him for a walk. This would get her moving and the dog moving. Suzanne was grasping the concept of small changes. Something is better than nothing.

My second topic was food. I had asked her to keep a food journal for the week before we met and based on that, her food choices were excellent. One dinner was roast pork, sauerkraut, mashed potatoes, green beans and ice cream cake. Another dinner was roast beef with mushrooms and gravy, pasta and broccoli and small biscotti. She's a self-admitted "foodie." She loves food and said she loves her kitchen and didn't want to give it up. I wouldn't take things away from her but we'll work on readjusting her thinking when it comes to all foods. Suzanne needs to have a healthier relationship with food.

I asked Suzanne to take "before" pictures of herself wearing a sports bra and bike pants. She handed the pictures to me and said, "That was the most humbling part. It's all about the belly. Lock those pictures away."

Suzanne talked about past diets. She'd lose weight relatively quickly then she'd go off the diets and regain the weight. I explained that she has to be careful with dieting because if she goes on a diet, she will go off a diet. I want her to make lifestyle changes, meaning what she does now, she'll do for the rest of her life. Having said that, our challenge was to find something Suzanne could realistically do forever.

"I have a real problem with waste. I will eat off the kids' plates so the food won't get thrown out." This was a red flag—eating someone else's food. "I'm a huge leftover person. My lunch could be the size of my dinner." Here was another red flag—eating a large lunch and then possibly eating a large dinner.

Suzanne doesn't like fruit but loves vegetables, so I wanted her to keep eating vegetables. If I asked her to start eating five fruits a day, she wouldn't, so this would not be a pleasant experience for her. We'll stay with what she likes and then slowly add fruit into her life.

We talked about fast food; thankfully Suzanne is not one to frequent those places. When parents tell me their child is overweight because he loves fast food and eats it several times a week, I ask, "Who drives the child to the restaurant?"

Suzanne is a serious dinner person; it's important to her. "Food is an event for me. I never miss a meal." Fortunately, she prepares healthful foods but there were more red flags. I have to find out why dinner is so important to her, why it's an event and why she never misses a meal. There is too much of an attachment to food and my goal will be to detach her. I have to be careful because Suzanne does love food and I want her to keep loving food—just not so much of it.

Suzanne wanted long-term success, not a quick fix like she's had on other diets. We talked about lunch and she had an interesting comment: "A frozen diet dinner would be done too fast." Suzanne likes to eat for a while.

As we talked, we developed two goals:

- Figure out strategies to avoid mindless eating (like while she is watching football games).
- Learn to throw things out rather than eat them, unless they would make a satisfying meal.

These two goals were the key to slowly detaching Suzanne from food.

The final topic was water; Suzanne needs to drink half her body weight in ounces of water. Since she is not doing this, she's to gradually add water into her life.

I talked about self-esteem and how it grows as my clients make subtle changes in their life. Even the dynamics of relationships change. Suzanne will experience this as she gains control of her life and her body.

We had an awesome conversation. Suzanne told me she has a plan to get started, so we both wrote these down:

- Get bike down; needs to go to the shop for repairs
- Dance class; call about it for her and Kris
- Put sneaks on when she gets home. (I want her to play with the kids—shoot hoops for 5-10 minutes, throw a football, ride bikes, do something, anything with them.)

We talked again about Suzanne's "before" photos and she said, "… humbling, motivating, eye-opening." I needed her to see what she looked like with few clothes on. Some clients are in denial and don't want to see what they look like. Some avoid mirrors. And, some choose not to weigh themselves because it's better not to know the number. But my feeling is that they have to 'fess up to the body they have. No more denial. For Suzanne, the photos are a starting point.

I explained to Suzanne how the brain fascinates me because she could exercise but she doesn't. We might spend a few sessions just talking and not exercising because we have to get her brain in order. Once we do that, she will have success from the neck down.

Saturday, January 6

Suzanne's Journal Notes …

"No breakfast, a good-size lunch, cheese stick for a snack then dinner with friends at 6:00 p.m. At 8:15 a.m., took a 4½-mile walk with Donna, Sue, Julie & Terry. 4:15 p.m., played 45 minutes of casual tennis with the family. A little sore from the abdominal exercises (how pathetic!)"

We'll need to address this "no breakfast" thing. It's the most important meal of the day and she can't skip it. She's getting friends to walk with her and she's getting the family involved by playing tennis with them. It doesn't matter what type of exercise it is; Suzanne just has to do something.

Tuesday, January 9

I saw Suzanne at a Women's Referral Network (WRN) luncheon and she was beaming. Maybe it was my imagination, but she sure looked happy. We've only met once but I can see her start to change. Suzanne told me she was 154 lbs.—three pounds lost. She's more aware of what she is eating, which resulted in a three-pound weight loss.

Wednesday, January 10

Suzanne's Journal Notes... ...

"At 8:00 p.m. I took a one-mile walk with my son Griffin; it was great to be with him and talk in the beautiful clear night."

Suzanne could have watched a television program or played a video game with her son, but she chose to walk with him. And they talked!

Friday, January 12

When we met, Suzanne announced, "The kids were getting on my nerves the other day so I sent them outside to play. Then I got on my coat and went outside with them." She could have stayed inside for solitude but she decided to go outside and play with them.

Suzanne felt victorious over last week's football game because she kept the food in the kitchen and out of the way of mindless eating. She actually threw out some crab dip and that was huge from the woman who didn't like to waste anything. Suzanne said she would have eaten four or five crackers to finish off the crab dip but she didn't, she threw it out!

Over the weekend Suzanne played 40 minutes of tennis with her son and said her heart was really pumping. She was so invigorated when she left the tennis court and is now starting to realize why the feeling is more important than the task itself.

At Tuesday's WRN luncheon, the speaker talked about goals and how we should have them, write them down and have a plan to achieve them. Suzanne asked if she should write down her goals, then said something very interesting. "I don't feel I'm ready to set a goal." We don't have to and can wait until she's ready, whenever that might be.

Suzanne has a weight goal for May but said, "135 pounds seems hard to reach by May." This sounded pretty aggressive, so we'll continue to take it slowly and see how her body responds. This isn't about winning a race; it's about helping Suzanne change her life. How long did it take her to get to 157 pounds? It was going to take us a while to get her weight down and keep it down.

I read to her the four goals she told me at our first meeting then she said, "The scale below 150 pounds would be huge."

I re-read her the goals and she wrote them in her exercise booklet:

- It's not really about weight; it's about being comfortable in my skin. I walk heavy and I feel heavy.
- Figure out how to fit fitness into my schedule on a regular basis and be excited about it.
- I want to start and keep it up—exercise.
- Life balance.

"There was a lot of awareness this week." Suzanne had broken her sweets habit last winter but then started eating sweets again. "I feel I made good choices this week. On Sunday and Monday I planned all of my meals for the week." Suzanne is learning how important planning is to her success. It would take about a year to gain total confidence because she has to go through all of the holidays, birthdays, tax season (she's a CPA), and so on, to see how she does. This is a journey.

At 10:00 a.m. we started with her weights routine. "I guess I need this too," she said with a frown as she looked down at the weights and exercise band. Unfortunately, some clients have this misperception that it's going to be too hard or too difficult to exercise. I want to make working out fun for Suzanne so she looks forward to it and I want her to feel successful in the process.

When doing a biceps exercise Suzanne said, "Get my boobs out of the way." I told her a story a golf professional told me at a golf lesson. The pro said the breasts are attached to your body; they're not going anywhere, so you might as well take them with you. It makes sense!

Suzanne commented that she doesn't want to look like a body builder. She doesn't have enough testosterone for that to happen.

Are the exercises do-able? "Definitely! This is perfect!" Suzanne saw that the exercises took a short period of time, so they wouldn't take a big chunk out of her day. If the exercises took too much time, chances are she wouldn't do them on a regular basis.

Saturday, January 13

Suzanne's Journal Notes ...

"Lunch at Jen's shower: diet cola, hot roast beef sandwich (didn't finish), quiche (didn't eat the crust), Caesar salad, a little chicken salad, and 2/3 of a piece of cake."

This shower could have been traumatic for Suzanne but we talked about it ahead of time and she went in with a plan. There was no mindless eating and she did the best she could with the choices she had. Positive changes are happening: she didn't finish the sandwich, she didn't eat the crust, she had just a taste of some things and she even had cake.

Monday, January 15

When we met, Suzanne commented that she was hungry, but it was only 11:45 a.m. She should eat a snack because I want her to eat about every three hours. Going from 8:00 a.m. to 1:00 p.m. is too long to wait, so she needs to add a healthful 100- to 200-calorie snack. If Suzanne were eating 1,500 calories a day, divided by five mini meals, she'd get

300 calories per meal. Then she said, "Please don't say 1,500 calories. I think I eat 3,000 a day."

We talked about her husband Kris not liking to take walks with her. Suzanne was seeing the walk as an exercise that would be good for him. I asked her to see the walk as time they could spend together. "Neck at the bridge!" Tell Kris that and he just might go on a walk.

Suzanne had a lot on her mind and was pleased knowing there are times we'll talk to get her through a situation. As long as she doesn't eat her problems, she's okay.

Tuesday, January 16

Suzanne sent an email:

> "Good morning Linda. I was 151 this morning—maybe it's real and not a fluke!? I haven't packed my lunch yet, but I am already thinking in healthy snack mode for mid-morning. Wow! I still can't thank you enough for the support, interest, knowledge and inspiration. I am in awe!"

Friday, January 19

I received an email from Suzanne with "Quick Question" in the subject line:

> "Good Morning Linda!
>
> "So far, so good this week. I wrote in my journal yesterday that I really had the munchies—maybe PMS!? Or...Ian was home sick, I did tons of housework in the morning and then was sporadically doing things after that—maybe I was a little bored?? Anyway, not too bad, and the family went to the local pizza shop for dinner. I had a small piece of vegetable stromboli—probably not the healthiest thing on the menu, but I didn't eat too much.
>
> "My question is...does it matter what time I do the exercises? The last three nights I have found myself doing them between 8:30 and 9:30 p.m. Is that too

late? I certainly haven't had any trouble sleeping after that. I am liking that time, because most of my 'duties' are finished by then."

PMS can definitely bring on the munchies, as can boredom. I explained that we want her to be able to eat with the family, so I'm glad she had the vegetable stromboli. The best part is that she hadn't eaten too much. As far as time of day to exercise, it doesn't matter when she exercises, just as long as she finds time to do it. Since it's not keeping her awake at night, evenings are fine.

Saturday, January 20

Suzanne's Journal Notes ...

"I did arms, push-ups and abs early today because Kris and I were off for our romantic getaway to Philly for the day/overnight with Tim and Rebecca. I knew my eating would not be too great. Lunch: 2:00 p.m., fast food burger (no fries!) and a diet cola—already off to a bad start. 3:30 p.m. Arrived in Philly, met up with friends and walked around shopping until around 6:00 p.m. 7:15 p.m. Cocktails—two glasses of champagne. Dinner: 8:30 p.m. Fitzwater Café (delicious and would go back in a heartbeat). We shared a bowl of their lobster bisque, antipasti with grilled eggplant, white beans, roasted peppers, fresh mozzarella cheese, two grilled shrimp (I shared), seafood risotto (appetizer for dinner and I didn't finish), but I had two small pieces of bread, Prosecco wine, water and a cappuccino for dessert. And then we were off dancing until 1:30 a.m. I had a few beers, water and a shot of something, and then we finally topped off the evening at the fast food place across from the hotel and I had two crispy chicken strips (I hope all the dancing helped!)."

It's exciting to see Suzanne sharing food, not finishing some of it and drinking water. Yes, the dancing helped burn off some of that meal. Then there are two ways to look at the late-night fast food stop: she shouldn't have been eating so late at night, especially crispy strips, which are fried, or she did an awesome job by not ordering a cheeseburger and fries. I chose the latter.

Monday, January 22

Since Suzanne likes playing tennis and her goal is to be excited about exercise, I suggested we attend a clinic. When she walked in, she looked the part in her cute tennis outfit. We had fun going through various drills then playing mini-games against other women. Suzanne commented that she was winded but she held her own. The hour-and-a-half clinic flew by and it was obvious she was enjoying herself. Perfect, here was another activity she could add to her exercise list.

Suzanne's Journal Notes ...

"Lesson learned: Last week I never did my weekly food planning and shopping; we 'made it through' with what was in the house. It made snacking very hard. Today, I made my plan for the week and it makes all the difference, especially in the healthiness of dinner. Now, next Monday I know I will be out of town at a client's office so I have to re-do my normal shopping schedule, but still get it done!"

I can't teach Suzanne these lessons. This is her journey and it's called "On-the-Job Training."

Thursday, January 25

I received this email from Suzanne:

"I loved the tennis and I really hope I can make more of the Mondays. I was supposed to go to a client's office in Doylestown today, but due to the possible ugly weather later, my co-worker decided not to go today, but I will have to go on Monday instead. I was really struggling with my schedule, because Monday is supposed to be my ½ day,

but I have to remember that it is busy season for me. I made the commitment to myself to give everything that I could into my health/training. I just have to continue to figure out how to fit it in. I am looking forward to lunch tomorrow. I feel like there is plenty to talk about…I can't always predict the work schedule during busy tax season, so how can I best schedule my workouts? I have done nothing other than the weights, legs, push-ups and abs for about two weeks (except for tennis and some awesome dancing Saturday night with Kris and friends). The weather has been a complete de-motivator for me. I think a good solution is the indoor bike stand, but I understand the stand will cost about $150 and I have to wait a couple weeks to buy one. I also have to look, but I think I still have an exercise step that I could dust off if there is a routine I could work on at home. Anyway, enough rambling, we can talk tomorrow. Thanks Linda!!!"

There was so much in her email that I didn't know where to begin:

- She loved tennis, so we've found something she'll be excited about.

- She's struggling with her schedule, wants to play tennis on Mondays but she's an accountant and they are going into tax season. Again, we've found an activity that sparks her interest enough to create a struggle in her mind. This means Suzanne is committed to the exercise part. If she were ho-hum about playing, then we'd have to find another activity.

- She made the commitment to herself to put everything that she could into her health and training. The intention is there. The motivation is there. But life gets in the way so we need to deal with that.

- Her comment about needing to figure out how to fit exercise in is key. I can't figure out anything for Suzanne. I can suggest that family members fold the laundry or set the table, but they might already be doing that.

- Suzanne is asking how she can best schedule her workouts. It doesn't matter when she works out during the day, but just that she carves out time to do it.

- I was sad when she said she's "done nothing other than the weights, legs, push-ups and abs for about two weeks." Nothing? She's done so much more than she was doing last month or even last year. Her expectation is too high and she's too new to this lifestyle change process. Her expectations need to be lowered to make her feel successful.

- The comment about "awesome dancing" with Kris is exciting. They like to dance, it counts as exercise and it's something she wants to do. Exercise doesn't mean spending an hour at the gym; it means doing some kind of activity where she's getting her body in motion more than she used to do.

- Cold weather and overcast days are de-motivators. Suzanne has to learn that the weather does not dictate her mood, only the activity she chooses to do.

- Because she cannot afford the bike stand for a few weeks, I suggested she look at cheaper options.

Her motivation cannot drop; not when she's doing so well. Meeting tomorrow will give her a much-needed shot in the arm.

Friday, January 26

At our weekly meeting, Suzanne talked about her daily exercises: "I haven't missed a day!" Originally, Suzanne said she couldn't do push-ups but she did eight, took a break, and then did eight more.

Each Sunday Suzanne plans for Monday's food shopping, so the need to plan has really sunk in.

"This might sound stupid, but at 7:30 p.m. there's nothing on TV to watch." Suzanne was thinking she could do a cardio workout during that time but not on their trampoline; after three bounces she needs to go into the bathroom…from having kids.

This morning Suzanne was 150.5 pounds. "I think the scale is a good thing for me, but I don't want to be obsessed." As we talked about sabotage and justifying the weight loss, Suzanne said, "I got overly confident Saturday morning. When I went to the fast food place I could have made more healthful choices, but I didn't, so I ate the burger instead of having a salad." We talked about using the scale versus using clothing to keep her accountable. When she took her jeans out of the dryer that morning, she realized she needed a belt. Now she is accountable to her jeans—the pair straight out of the dryer.

"I feel really good about the legs, abs and arms exercises. It's almost a habit."

Suzanne is a *Cooking Light* magazine fan. She loves to make recipes from the magazine and commented on knowing how many calories were in a particular recipe. She still needs to watch the portions because sometimes the calories are for a very small serving, by her standards. I made a note to give her one of my favorite calorie-counting books, *The CalorieKing Calorie, Fat & Carbohydrate Counter* by Allan Borushek. Just as I was writing it down, she said, "I don't ever want to count calories." I told her about the book and how it could be a guide for her. "It will be hard. I love food so much." Because of her love for food, smaller portions will be a key to her success.

Our meetings had been at a studio or restaurant, but now I wanted to meet at her house. She informed me that the house is not set up to exercise, so we talked about setting it up, possibly in the basement. On my napkin I drew a square and said this will be an area she claims as her own. I talked about having a TV down there or a CD or DVD player, but she said she wouldn't do two things at once—watch TV and exercise. In the case of her favorite show—"24," she has to give it her undivided attention. "Exercising at 7:30 p.m. will make me more productive for the rest of the evening."

"The boys each have their own room. Kris has his chair and I don't have my own room or space. I want to put my step out and leave it out. The kids leave their Lego® building blocks out, so I want to leave my toys out."

On my napkin, in the space that was roped off for her, I drew a picture of a bike and a step.

She felt Kris would want her exercise equipment in the corner by the drafty door. I asked if this would motivate her to go into the basement—exercising by a drafty door. "No!" So we need to find another place for her exercise space. We talked about the big sofa and I suggested moving it. "This will be the first thing that impacts the family."

I explained that the dynamics of relationships could change, so her husband, family and friends might not like me or might not like the change in Suzanne. These people are used to having Suzanne a certain way and then she starts acting differently. She had not talked to Kris about her becoming thinner and the impact it will have on him so she needs to, to gain his support. Suzanne needs to tell him she's not going to be biking in the basement for an hour. "That's not going to happen!" Kris doesn't know that so she needs to reassure him and her boys about her intentions.

Suzanne is "psyched" about making space in the basement for her exercise equipment. Recently, she had gone over to Mary's house and noticed Mary had space in her home to call her own. Suzanne said, "I remembered thinking that I didn't know how to get it—space."

Suzanne is to let me know if she's ready or when she's ready to get more exercises. The exercises have become a daily part of her life and they need to stay that way. This journey is on her timetable, not mine.

Saturday, January 27

Suzanne's Journal Notes ...

"4:00 p.m. My first bike ride in a long time. Rode over to Mom's house with my son KJ and then did the Hershey's Mill loop. I only got stuck on one hill and boy, did my legs shake when I got off. But it really felt good. I want to feel more secure on my bike, and I love the wind in my face and of course, being with KJ."

What a great journal entry! We have worked together only 27 days and I know Suzanne will achieve her goals sooner than she thinks.

Tuesday, January 30

Suzanne sent an email:

> "The space is not cleaned out yet, but I have a plan for where my exercise space will be. I have told Kris about it and didn't really get any objections. I found my step; now I just have to dust it off. I won't have the bike stand by Thursday, but my goal is to have the step in place and the Lego blocks moved over to their allotted space! Today I am feeling heavy for some reason. My weight has stayed right at 151. I know I have significantly reduced my eating quantities and the sweets, so I am trusting that I just have to keep it up and maybe reduce even further. I'll see you Thursday. Stay warm! Suz
>
> "P.S. I walked with my girlfriend last Sunday afternoon. The snow started and it was a beautiful time to be outside."

Wednesday, January 31

If January is an indicator of how the rest of our time together is going to go, we're in for an awesome journey. When Suzanne and I first met, she set goals, which let her know what she wanted. Through the month she learned the importance of having fun while exercising, dealt with expectations that were too high, found out when to exercise and started to create her own space…exercise space. Suzanne is mindful of her eating and she's exercising on a daily basis. These small changes are sinking in and are becoming part of her life.

To Do:

1. Find an accountability partner. Make sure it is someone you trust and someone who knows what he or she is doing.

2. Set goals

3. Keep a journal of everything you eat and drink

4. Exercise daily, even if it's only 10 minutes

February:
Creating Habits with Little Time

Thursday, February 1

I went to what I thought was Suzanne's address, but it didn't look like it could be her house. Since no one answered the doorbell, I drove down the street. Ah, there it was—a beautiful, well-kept, nicely manicured house with a pretty wreath on the front door.

I met Tucker the dog and learned that he had been a Christmas gift to one of Suzanne's sons. Suzanne said it had been her best Christmas on record because of how excited her son was to have a puppy. She commented about her shins hurting from walking Tucker yesterday; rather, he walked her.

Her official weight was 150 pounds; seven pounds lost in January. We talked about Suzanne not being obsessed with the scale, but then she admitted, "The scale is a motivator."

I asked her to save some January clothes and she said, "I can't imagine getting rid of any." I was talking about her 157-pound clothes. If she's having a day when she doesn't think she's lost weight, she can put on those jeans—the ones that now need a belt—and they will let her know her progress.

We discussed the need for Suzanne to allow herself to eat and drink anything she wants, in moderation. Giving her permission takes the mystery out of foods she might be trying to avoid.

She shared a story about moderation: "I could have had half the sleeve of cookies, but instead I had the 100-calorie pack." Excellent!

Suzanne is a member of the Clean Plate or Eat-It-All-Club, which means what she packs for lunch is what she eats for lunch. We're slowly trying to break her of this habit and it is happening. "Really huge for me—I didn't eat the yogurt I packed."

Suzanne wanted to know more about the "Eat until you're full" mentality. Some clients, when their stomach grumbles from hunger, are feeling lonely or empty so they eat till they have a full feeling, even if it means overeating. For other clients, it's purely a physical feeling so they eat till they feel full. These clients are in the minority. So far, Suzanne doesn't seem to be an emotional eater. This means she's going to have to learn to listen to her body and stop eating when she's full. She said, "Eating muesli cereal for breakfast fills me up. It's the Linda way, catch it before you're starving." Right. Suzanne shouldn't wait till she's ravenous because then she might eat too much.

"I'm feeling a little bit of guilt—no cardio since the weekend." This statement said it all; she wants to exercise. Suzanne said she's doing fine with her new lifestyle changes and feels it is something she can live with.

"I love food!" Yes, she has mentioned that before.

Suzanne said years ago she bought candy from someone who was doing a fundraiser. She had the candy in her desk for months and would treat herself to a few pieces each day. This disciplined behavior will help her succeed with weight loss; she does not binge, so portion size will be important.

I asked Suzanne to take photos on February 4. "Oh gosh, really? I have to put the same thing on? I was so depressed when I did it the last time. Do you think there's a change?" I answered yes, because she's lost seven pounds and is working out daily.

I gave her a copy of the calorie, fat & carbohydrate counter book. Since Suzanne doesn't want to count calories, she's going to use this book as a reference. It will help her with choices, like the time she ordered a Caesar salad thinking it is a healthful choice when in fact it is not.

"I thought this was big for me. If you look at my journal, on Saturday it looks like I ate half the house but I didn't. I had a bite of dessert and didn't want it. I enjoyed the conversation, yet I was staring at food. I remembered the conversation with our company, when in the past I couldn't remember what we talked about. Before I only remembered the food."

Suzanne doesn't eat a lot of bread, which is fine. The kids like white potatoes and she likes sweet potatoes, which are better for her.

"Your approach is brilliant so far!" Suzanne was referring to my suggestion that she watch what she eats and drinks and that she exercise daily. This is a slow journey, not a sprint.

Referencing her new calorie book, Suzanne said, "I'm such a moron. I should have gone for the smaller burger." She had just learned that the big burger contains 800 calories and the smaller one has half that.

"Let me see how much damage I did with those two chicken strips." Suzanne was pleased with their calorie count, so I asked about the fat content. "I don't know what that means yet." I explained that if something is high in calories, it's typically high in fat. One of her goals is to lose weight so she needs to lower her calories, which will help lower the fat. The big and small burgers are perfect examples—the latter had half the calories and half the fat.

We talked about chicken, which is both a low-fat and low-calorie choice. If Suzanne eats too much chicken, even though it's low-fat, it still has calories and could make her gain weight. "I'm trying to watch portion sizes."

On Saturday evening two couples will be coming over to her house to plan their trip to Italy. Suzanne said she would have healthful foods available to eat. Planning is another key to her losing weight.

We stood near the huge Lego layout, but as Suzanne said, she has boys who still play with them, so the Lego blocks need to stay. It's a great idea to keep the boys busy with something other than the television or video games.

Suzanne showed me her daily routine without referring to notes, which let me know she had it memorized. Several times she asked, "Am I passing?"

Yes, she was. During an exercise she said, "I love this one." I'm glad to hear she likes an exercise. I about fell over when she asked, "Want to add any?" Not yet, but I love her enthusiasm. Her push-up form was awesome and she proudly said, "Go girl!"

Suzanne hasn't stepped in five years. I took her through several moves and hearing her breathing on some of them told me she really did need to do cardio work. Moves and patterns were coming back to her. "Oh, I remember all this." She did great and picked it up immediately. This new step routine took four minutes and 22 seconds and it was her choice to do it twice. "I'm losing my underwear. That might be too much information for you."

While taking a break Suzanne expressed some concerns about Kris and his job. I kept listening to hear if this might impact her exercising or eating. So far, she was okay.

We spent over an hour together; "Show Suzanne Stretches" was on my checklist but we were out of time. "Is there anything else?" I asked. "Stretches." Wow, we're thinking alike, so I showed her some.

During the triceps stretch Suzanne exclaimed, "Oh, I love this one!" And when we did the chest stretch she said, "This looks like a good one for your posture."

"Even if I lose a pound every two weeks, by the end of the year that's a lot of weight." Yes, it is.

As I was leaving Suzanne's house, I thought about our being together for only a month. I can't wait to see what happens to her in these next few months!

Sunday, February 4

Suzanne's Journal Notes ...

"Super Bowl Sunday! 1:00 p.m., huge walk with Carol and Caitlin (two very good friends), both very thin and have had fitness as a daily priority in their lives forever. I have

> *walked with them before and it is hard for me. They walk very fast. We walked Caitlin's route, which is somewhere between five and six miles on the streets (with plenty of hills!). I dressed very warm for the cold weather and I was plenty warm. It was a beautiful winter day. And I felt great when we were finished."*

Good for Suzanne; she didn't use the nine-degree wind chill as an excuse not to exercise and she was able to keep up with her fit friends. Her self-confidence is building!

According to her journal, she could have had lots of junk food on Super Bowl Sunday but chose not to.

Tuesday, February 6

> *"Hi Linda, I woke up this morning and realized that we don't have a time to get together on the calendar for this week. We could meet for coffee or lunch.*
>
> *"So far the week has been great. I weighed in Monday morning at 150. I went back over my journal and realized that I have been 151 and 152 the last two weeks on Monday and 150 and 151 on Friday of the same week. If my pattern stays true, I should be 149 by Friday. That would be HUGE milestone for me."*

This email is awesome for two reasons: she wants to meet with me (when a client isn't sticking to her program, she will avoid me) and she's figuring out a weight pattern. I asked her to leave a message on my cell phone when she hits the 140s.

Friday, February 9

I was disappointed that my morning appointment was cancelled, so I decided to use the time to do paperwork. Suddenly, my phone rang and it was a very happy-sounding Suzanne. "I'm calling to tell you I hit the 149 mark! The needle really was at 149. I'll see you at 12:30 p.m., but that's my good morning news!" Our conversation was just a few minutes long but I was glad my earlier appointment had been cancelled so I could talk with Suzanne.

After we hung up, I kept thinking about what was making Suzanne succeed. Is it because she's a goal-oriented person who has a desire to achieve things? She is not going to a gym or working out for an hour each day. She's not sacrificing time with her family to achieve her goals. She hasn't given up her kitchen or her love for food. What she has done is plan things, work out daily (if only for ten to twenty minutes), and be aware.

Suzanne's journey is about building a strong mind and a strong body. She is more confident and I guarantee she will not go back to 157 pounds or the way she used to be. Suzanne likes how she's feeling now. It is the taste of success. She is creating balance in her life.

I was already at the restaurant when Suzanne arrived. She was excited about her weight but said she put too much pressure on herself. She couldn't sleep this morning because she was going to weigh in. We'll have to work on less emphasis on the scale.

At the table Suzanne didn't dig right into her meal as she had in the past. She waited because we were talking. The shift is slowly moving away from the food to the conversation.

We put her pictures on the table and looked at each view from last month versus this month. Yes, there was a slight difference.

Suzanne asked about taking measurements but I suggested letting her jeans do the measuring—they need a belt because they are too loose. With measurements, if we don't get the exact same spot on each body part and the inches go up, this will not motivate Suzanne. We could do her stomach by starting the tape on her belly button. This would ensure that we have the same spot each time. I'll let her decide.

She was pleased to be 150 pounds last Friday and still 150 pounds this past Monday because, "It was not the best weekend."

I asked Suzanne why she has been successful. "I'm paying attention." I said she had lost seven pounds and she corrected me because today it's eight pounds.

Suzanne doesn't have an indoor bike stand yet. It's too cold outside to get her bike in the car then take it to a bike shop. She wants to test the stand to make sure she's comfortable with it.

"This might sound strange, but something as basic as changing clothes makes a difference in what I do—it takes time to change clothes." Suzanne explained that she changes clothes to go to work, changes clothes to go to a church meeting, and then changes clothes to work out. One evening she did the step routine in slippers because, "walking upstairs might not allow me to get back downstairs again." We laughed and I was okay with the slippers on occasion but don't want her walking with her fitness friends in them.

She likes meeting weekly but warned me it might get harder as we get into tax season. We'll do the best we can, even if it's a 30-minute coffee break each week to check in.

Suzanne shared a "minor victory" with me. She had packed her lunch and taken it to work, then Kris called wanting to go out to eat, so they did. The victory was that she saved this lunch. The next day, another "minor victory" was not eating all that she had packed in one sitting, as she normally would do—she saved some of the meal till later in the day.

We talked about meeting weekly versus monthly. "I wouldn't be as aware of the little things if we met monthly. Meeting with you weekly keeps me on track. You're giving me these awesome tools. I'm not doing this for you, except for the pictures, but I understand why you want the pictures."

I asked if our working together has been hard and she said "No! This has not been painful at all. I don't feel deprived or overworked. But how long till I have to increase my activity or decrease my food?" This is a very common question and I explained to Suzanne that she's like a snow-woman, melting away the pounds. Currently, this is not the right weight for her, because her body is responding to the amount of food and exercise she's giving it. Her body will tell us when it's reached its limit by slowing down the weight-loss process. If she gets into tax season but doesn't have time to exercise or plan meals like she's doing now, she'll have to maintain her weight till she has time to do the above. This really is all about timing and planning.

Suzanne emailed Kris that she was 149 pounds. "It will take awhile till he takes this seriously. I deserve not to be taken seriously right now because I've started and stopped on numerous occasions."

Kris appreciates Suzanne's delicious home-cooked meals. She said her dad had heart issues and her mom cooked healthfully, but her dad didn't appreciate it…. he'd go out and have kielbasa and a beer for lunch. Having Kris cooperate is important to Suzanne's success.

Suzanne and I talked about working together through May. Ideally, I'd like to work with her for a year so we can go through holidays, birthdays, vacations and so on. Each event is an opportunity to make sure Suzanne is on track and stays on track.

"The goal was not about losing weight. The long-term success is so much more important to me than the immediate gratification." What a profound statement. Suzanne understands that this is not about immediate gratification or immediate results; this journey is about creating healthy habits for life.

Suzanne is able to exercise after dinner and after the boys' homework is done. She's learning about balance and priorities and making time for herself. She's also learning what works best for her.

Suzanne asked about the people who surround her—how important are they? This was an excellent question. If her fitness friends wanted to drink beer and eat junk food after a walk, that would be counterproductive. The people around her can motivate or hinder her, so she should choose them wisely. What is Suzanne trying to achieve? This journey is about her, not about other people. She needs to be strong enough mentally to stand up to the pressures of others. She must have been reading my mind. "I'm not in the mood to have six beers when we go out this evening because I'm having a good day." Suzanne is getting mentally strong!

In general, does she feel better about herself? "Yes. Before I felt less confident professionally. Now I'm feeling more confident. Baby steps. I had an evaluation at work and held my ground. I also had an international conference call, dialed in, understood all the different accents and did fine. In the past, I would have been hesitant about both of these."

One of Suzanne's goals is to do activities with her children and it has happened. Proudly she said, "KJ asked if we were going to do push-ups together."

As we were leaving the restaurant, Suzanne actually left some of her meal and soda. It is sinking in that she doesn't have to finish everything. Yes, it will go to waste, but it's better than being on her waist.

Sunday, February 11

Suzanne's Journal Notes ...

"I felt thinner today. I put on my non-fat pants and a sweater I haven't worn for quite a while and went to church. I had room in the pants, and the sweater even made me look like I had a waist. I feel great. I am a little bummed I did not get an outside activity in today. The weather was certainly nice enough for a walk, but I just couldn't work out the timing. I have been thinking about my conversation with Linda. She asked me why I thought I was being successful so far. I'm not sure. I know I started this very unsure if I could do it. I wasn't even as motivated as I thought I should have been. I did feel a strong obligation to Linda because she offered to work with me for five months. But then she made getting started so doable. From that point on, my confidence in my own ability to work toward my goals seemed possible."

Friday, February 16

Suzanne's Journal Notes ...

"149 lbs.—crap! I went from the euphoria last Friday of thinking I could conquer the world to feeling a little less than that today. I swear I think it is hormones. I also think that is has to do with control for me. It started out with a funeral on Monday that messed up the schedule (not that I would have been any place else!). Tuesday the kids were dismissed early from school because of the weather, so I packed up work and went home, but got no work done. Wednesday, there was no school for the kids. No, I did not do any shoveling, sledding or general frolicking in the snow. I stayed in my slippers all day until I went to the deck to grill pork chops. I only got a few hours of billable work done. Thursday the kids had a two-hour delay and then I had a report card committee meeting at 1:00 p.m., so it didn't make sense to go to the office. I got a couple hours of work done in the morning, but now here it is Friday and my billable hours are awful. I did, however, manage to get the sheets all washed and the rest of the laundry done, and the house is actually in pretty good order.

"I didn't miss my legs/arms, push-ups or abs exercises so that is a positive. And I did manage to make a few good food choices this week. I think I just made my portions too big again. Well, it's a new day and a new opportunity to be productive here at work and make healthy choices. I feel better already."

Because there was some doubt in Suzanne's journal entry, I wanted to put things into perspective for her. I sent her an email saying she's doing an outstanding job, then listed what she's accomplished: lost eight pounds, did 30 push-ups one night, went through the step routine a record four times for a total of 23 minutes, has kept a daily journal since January 1, has exercised daily, is planning meals and watching portions.

Suzanne responded:

> *"Linda, Thank you so much for the pick-me-up. I truly am feeling better. I think I just needed to get out of my house and start working on the work I didn't get done this week. Plus, we were entertaining and I am cooking both Saturday and Sunday nights, so I think I was feeling overwhelmed about everything I have to do. It's all good, and I am looking forward to getting together next week. Hopefully, it will be a more predictable week!"*

Suzanne needs to feel the high of last Friday and the low of this Friday. Her journey has a lot to do with feelings. We don't talk about exercise that much—it's a sidebar.

Wednesday, February 21

Suzanne gave me a tour of her gorgeous home. They added on to the house so the kitchen is huge. "We use it hard," she said of the kitchen and house, which could be in a decorator magazine.

There were adorable family pictures on the wall and she showed me their Christmas photo—taken on the beach—of this attractive-looking group.

"It has been a tough, tough, tough food weekend. I was 150 pounds Monday and knew I would be because of entertaining friends over the weekend. I was 149 pounds last Wednesday and I need to get serious."

The snowy weather has kept Suzanne inside and is making her feel claustrophobic "I feel very closed in. I was thinking about taking a walk after you left but I like to walk with someone."

"Saturday I worked in the morning, came home to straighten up the house, cooked like a loon, had company then did my exercises at midnight. Tonight is not the night that I am not going to do my exercises. Maybe if I had the flu, but I don't."

We went through Suzanne's new exercises and she did fine. She's strengthening all different muscles and is avoiding the repetition of just walking or riding her bike. For the exercises, I asked that she do the same number of repetitions on each side because we're continuing to work on muscle balance. She's to avoid doing more repetitions on her stronger side. "I'm an accountant—I couldn't possibly do that."

During the triceps exercise she commented about her left arm, "Oh, my gosh, my arm is shaking. My left is definitely not as strong. I remember talking about muscle imbalance a few weeks ago, so now I pour the laundry detergent with my left hand."

"You're going to take away my favorite abs exercise?" No, if Suzanne likes something, she will be motivated to keep doing it.

To be as efficient as possible with the time she has, every exercise should have a purpose and some exercises would be harder than others. "Harder didn't necessarily mean that it took more time, which is a good thing." This was an interesting comment because Suzanne originally equated harder with taking more time.

After going through all of the new exercises I asked Suzanne if she could imagine doing 16 repetitions of each. "Not today."

"I can do these daily. Beautiful!"

Thursday, February 22

Suzanne's Journal Notes ...

"148 lbs.! 8:30 p.m., Twenty-four minutes on the step (four times through routine), 20 of the new push-ups, new abs routine and arms. I did the push-ups and abs with my son KJ. It was a lot of fun doing it together. He was playing a game on the computer while I was on the step. He said he likes the rhythm of my feet during the step routine. It felt good tonight. I was sweating when I was finished."

Friday, February 23

Suzanne's Journal Notes ...

"149 lbs.—boo hoo! Even though the weight went back up, now I know I can get it back down to 148. It has been a good week. I have felt like I got a lot of work done at the office and the house is in pretty good shape. I am ready for the weekend. We have a really special dinner at a friend's house on Saturday night. It is sort of a wine-tasting (we're doing South African wines) but the hosts pair the food with the wine and I know it will be something really great, so portion control may be difficult. Although, on the positive side, it won't be junk food—all fresh ingredients—so it already is better for me than a night at a fast food restaurant!"

Saturday, February 24

Suzanne's Journal Notes ...

"Dinner: 7:30 p.m., our much-anticipated wine dinner with Laura and Tim. It was fabulous! We had a five-course dinner with a different wine with each course, and the theme of the wine was South African wines. And I had everything. The portions weren't huge, and I certainly didn't have seconds on anything, but I ate everything that was served. I don't know if I could ever get to the point that I wouldn't eat everything in this circumstance. The company was marvelous. Kris and I knew the hosts and I knew Lisa, but the other five guests were all new friends for us. We laughed the entire night. I was so glad I exercised before we went out! We didn't leave until about 1:30 a.m.!"

Why is Suzanne having such success on her journey? In anticipation of a late night, she did her daily exercises before going out. Then, she ate what she wanted, watched her portions and didn't go back for seconds.

Sunday, February 25

Suzanne's Journal Notes ...

"6:00 p.m., five times through the step routine and I jogged in the beginning and hopped some, just trying to get my heart rate up a little more and a little faster. It really worked. I did some serious sweating. I did 40 push-ups (with a break in between) and the abs.

"During the Oscars show I had leftover kettle popcorn that Ian had made much earlier and had been just sitting on the island. Now that tops my stupid eating since I started this in January—it wasn't even good. It was cold—but it was still sitting there. I obviously know the solution to the problem—throw the leftover cold stale popcorn in the trash!!!! Oh, and at least I had water! I had planned on getting some computer work done during the Oscars. I thought it would be the perfect time to catch up since I could do it and still enjoy the show. But as it turned out, I was too lazy (or tired from the night before) to get motivated to do anything. I think I was mad at myself for not doing anything (and I was bored) so I ate the popcorn. I know it's not the end of the world and I did a great job of exercising, but my mood was down the next day because the stuff I wanted to get done—and didn't—still remained un-done!"

Because Suzanne is journaling, she is starting to pick up on things: she was bored so she ended up eating stale popcorn. She has to learn these lessons so she can respond differently the next time, like throwing out the kettle popcorn.

Wednesday, February 28

I got to Suzanne's house early, so I drove around the neighborhood. It's hilly, which means she's getting a good workout while walking.

Right away she told me about a phone call she had received. Friends were coming over this evening and they want to go out for a cheese steak. "Dilemma—what do I eat?" We sent Suzanne into the evening with a plan: have a small piece of anything they ordered plus a salad. This allows her to be part of the gang, not feel deprived and still stay on track.

"I'm bummed about my weight. Is it muscle?" Her new set point is 150 pounds, not 157 and her slight increase in weight is not muscle. "Damn!"

"Since this whole thing started, I've been comfortable and made healthy choices." Then Suzanne used the word "failure" and said she'd have to "step it up." Failure is negative but her desire to "step it up" is positive.

Suzanne is to start keeping track of her daily water consumption and drink half her body weight in ounces.

Does she have March goals? "I'm going to have a weight goal, which is shocking me because I didn't want this to be about weight. Now I'm afraid! But here is my goal: 146 pounds. I can lose a pound a week till the end of the month." She talked about how she'll do this; she'll increase her cardio.

"This may sound trivial, but I want to give up chocolate at the office." Suzanne was reading the look on my face because she followed this up with, "I know I'm depriving myself but I eat them at the office because the candies are there. When I'm at home, I eat chocolate because I want it."

We talked about our working together. "It hasn't been hard. I haven't pushed myself; I've just eaten less food." Now Suzanne is realizing that to get to her ultimate goals, she is going to have to start pushing herself a little bit.

She wrote down her March goals:
- To be 146 pounds by Puerto Rico, the end of the month
- To drink 75 ounces of water a day
- No chocolate at the office

Suzanne is going into her busy tax season at work and wasn't sure how to incorporate cardio into her day. I suggested walking and she said, "I've called my walking friends, but they haven't called back." Again, she was reading my facial expression, "I know… I could walk by myself."

She needs to really watch her food portions. She agreed but didn't think she could do it. We'll have to work on that thinking.

I didn't want Suzanne to feel self-conscious the next time we went out to eat but I felt I needed to share this with her. There was such a difference from the first time we met for lunch, when she seemed interested in the food, versus the second time, when there was much less of an interest. She explained, "The first time we met for lunch, I was worked up that you didn't eat." Because we've discussed this, Suzanne is realizing that the focus is more on the person and conversation and less on the food.

How is she feeling during all that we've discussed so far? "Good, but I'm hungry and I don't like that feeling." I explained, as I had earlier in the month, that some clients don't like the hungry feeling because it makes them feel lonely or sad. She couldn't relate to that, which reinforces my thought that Suzanne is not an emotional eater.

"It's very inspirational to get together with you. You've snuck it in there—45 minutes of exercising. It's more than the five minutes a day like we started with, and it's fun!"

"I feel like I gave you a brain dump." It's okay because her journey isn't just about losing weight or exercising. It's about creating lifestyle changes.

"I don't find the new tripod push-ups any harder. They're not harder." She's doing them shallow, so I had her take her body almost to the floor. When she got there, she just lay there laughing and didn't get back up. Suzanne agreed to do shallow push-ups till she gets stronger.

If she's going to start jogging on the step, I reminded her about wearing two sports bras for support. She commented about being sore after doing the new exercises. This is why we have to keep changing her exercises, to challenge her body.

Suzanne told me an interesting story about last month's weekend with friends in Philadelphia. She couldn't understand why her friends packed workout clothes and went a day early to work out. Suzanne said, "Who packs their workout clothes? And now I'm thinking about it for Puerto Rico! I'll pack this exercise band and will try to find room in my luggage for sneakers. They might have a gym. We'll be eating out three times a day with a buffet breakfast."

I hugged her goodbye and swear I got a big bear hug back.

In our second month together, Suzanne learned that either the scale or her clothes would be a motivator. She was focusing on the conversation instead of food. The weather outside was not an excuse; she walked with her fit friends on a day with a wind chill of nine degrees. Success was coming from planning, working out and paying attention to what she was doing. She was getting stronger at home and at work. She experienced a shift in thinking.

To Do:

1. Continue to keep your journal

2. Change up the exercises

3. Look back at your progress

March:

A Month of Firsts

Friday, March 2

Suzanne's Journal Notes ...

"I am supposed to be working, but I thought it was time for another reality check and find out about how many calories I am eating. So I used Linda's book and looked up yesterday's food. It totals 1,400 calories, which is better than I expected. I have some leftover blueberries that I would like to make into some muffins or something. I went online to the Food Network's recipe bank and found a delicious-sounding scone recipe, but I decided to try and figure out the calories before I made them. Well, the scones would be 424 calories apiece. I obviously have a lot to learn about calories because I didn't think they could be that bad. Needless to say, I am not making that recipe."

Monday, March 5

I had emailed Suzanne Wednesday afternoon about scheduling our next meeting, but didn't hear back from her till this morning:

"Good Morning Linda, I am sorry for the delay in getting back to you. Ian was sick last Thursday & Friday, so I wasn't at the office and therefore couldn't get my schedule coordinated. I would prefer the Thursday at 8:00 a.m. time. I will just need five minutes at about 8:30 a.m. to get Ian to the bus stop. Saturdays are tough right now between being at the office and having a houseful at home. So if Thursday is still okay, please confirm.

"Kris took my pictures this morning and he actually commented that he could see a difference and was openly very proud of me. It felt great. So the picture thing wasn't quite as horrible as before. I was also under the weather over the weekend, so I was a little off my game. I guess the only positive note about that is that I have not eaten with my normal vigor! I really feel thinner today and I can see and feel it in my pants! Since we met last week I have done some calorie counting and referencing the book you gave me and it has been quite educational. See you Thursday (I hope). Suz"

Tuesday, March 6

An email came this afternoon:

"Hi Linda, I have two questions: 1. What should be my targeted daily calorie count? 2. Does iced tea count toward my water or only water and seltzer? I have been trying to pay a little more attention to my calorie intake. I was 148 this morning and had a really good workout last night. I really wish it would warm up! I am looking forward to getting together on Thursday."

Suzanne's calorie count should be around 1,500-1,700 calories a day and iced tea doesn't count toward her water. Since the forecast is for snow Wednesday, I reminded her that playing in the snow counts as exercise.

Thursday, March 8

When I got to Suzanne's house, Ian let me in and immediately informed me that he is going to be seven next month, three days before Easter. Just as important as his birthday is the fact that he likes the big chocolate Easter bunnies. Suzanne chimed in that she likes anything chocolate, anything with peanut butter in it, and Peeps—stale Peeps. We all went to the basement and Suzanne apologized for the mess of Lego building blocks.

"The infamous envelope," she said as she handed me her photos. We spread them out and compared them to the January photos—157 pounds versus 148 pounds. We noticed a difference in her stomach and back.

Fortunately, Suzanne isn't weighing herself as often and is "less obsessive."

We talked about moving the extra dinner food off the center of the table and onto the island or keeping it on the stove. She'll ask Kris about that because he's trying to cut back, too. I explained that this would help avoid the temptation of reaching and scooping versus having to get up to get a second helping. She added that she's more aware of calories now.

We talked about Goal #1—being 146 pounds by the end of March. "I'm gonna get it. I think I can. I think we're on track."

Goal # 2 is to drink 75 ounces of water daily. "I'm definitely doing that." Suzanne has to go to the bathroom all the time, which is common when getting used to drinking this much water.

How is she doing with Goal #3—to not eat chocolate at work? "Fine, but yesterday was really hard because I wasn't satisfied with my lunch. I brushed my teeth and that helped."

Suzanne had been prepared to have leftovers for dinner when Kris called to say he wanted to go out to eat. When they got to the restaurant, she said, "I really worked hard on the menu. Six months ago I would have had the lasagna and eaten the whole thing."

She's spending more time in the calorie book—her choice. Suzanne told me the blueberry scone story and how she figured out the calories then threw out the recipe. "You're sneakily getting me to count calories and do things I wouldn't and didn't want to do." She figured she had 1,740 calories one day and I had given her a range of 1,500 to 1,700. I haven't asked Suzanne to count calories, so the desire to do so is coming from her.

I explained that 1,500 calories a day, divided by five meals, would make each meal about 300 calories. This gives Suzanne a number to visualize. Eating her 70-calorie string cheese allows her to have more calories at other times throughout the day.

"I love a raisin bagel with peanut butter but there's 190 calories in two tablespoons of peanut butter." We're not taking food or the pleasure of food away from Suzanne; she just needs to be aware of the choices she is making.

Suzanne took a break to take Ian out to the bus stop then we went back to her goals. Goal #4 is to exercise five times a week for 15 minutes, cardio. "At least—and I'm ready for a new step routine."

My Goal #5 is portion control. "I think I have been. I definitely feel better and am more aware of calories."

Is this a lifestyle Suzanne can live with for the rest of her life? "Yes, but I had a fleeting moment last night while doing cardio. I asked myself, 'Will I have to do cardio every day for the rest of my life?'" I said she wouldn't and explained that we're getting her down to a size she wants to be then we'll concentrate on maintenance.

Suzanne said this snowy time of year is difficult for exercising outside because it's too slushy to bike and too cold to walk. She has indoor and outdoor activities, so she gets to choose which she wants to do.

"I still want to get my indoor bike holder." She doesn't want to exercise outside in the oppressive heat but doesn't like the cold; when she buys the holder is up to her.

We were done asking each other questions so we went through the step routine. "It's hard to step during American Idol." I showed her Fast Feet, which is a quick-step going clockwise around the step. "I'm gonna hate you for that." Suzanne calls them Hurry Ups. After doing four sets of eight repetitions I could hear a tiny breath. "You're going to make me go the other way, aren't you?" Yes, and she's catching on to my thinking.

I had her march on the top of the step then alternate a double lunge (tap back) for eight repetitions, and then alternate single lunges for two sets of eight. "My heiny's gonna like that one. Oh, my gosh!"

"Left Fast Feet times four?" "Yes." After two minutes of stepping I could hear her breathing so I asked about her heart rate. "It's good. It's up.

I love it!" I could still hear her breathing at the three-and-a-half-minute mark. Her form was excellent. "Thanks!"

The step routine took a total of seven minutes. Suzanne said her fitness friend, Carolyn is, "light on her feet" and I said someday she will be, too.

I have a few more things to share with Suzanne and she said, "Cardio?" No. "You're gonna bring me a big ball, aren't you?" Again, Suzanne was reading my mind because I am bringing her a ball. She talked about seeing the ball commercials on TV and liking the peoples' abs. "I know I won't have those abs because of my stomach."

Suzanne shared a touching story with me, one money can't buy. As she was doing push-ups, her oldest son, KJ, said, "Mom, I'm just in time." After they did push-ups, Suzanne said, "Okay, abs," and they did abdominal exercises together. "KJ's so proud of me! He'll go in and tell his gym teacher what his mom is doing exercise-wise."

Suzanne is realizing why exercises have to be changed on a regular basis. Muscles will get used to what she's doing and eventually won't respond as they should. Her breathing and her muscles are reacting to the new moves.

As she was writing down the moves, she asked, "How many of your appointments include a workout for you? Some day we'll do a workout?" Not all appointments include a workout and yes; we will be doing a workout when she's ready.

She hugged me hi and I hugged her bye. They are long hugs; sometimes words just can't fully express how appreciative she is.

"Tomorrow's scale day and we'll see what happens."

Friday, March 9

Suzanne sent me an email:

> "Good Morning Linda. Well, I may have to rethink one of my goals because…I was 146 this morning!!!!!!! I jumped

up and down on the scale to make sure and it kept saying the same weight. I hope I am not going to kick myself, but when I set the weight goal, I really wanted to set it at 145, but I was feeling a little unsure about whether the scale was going to start moving down again, so I thought 146 would still be good (and it is!), but 145 sounds even better. I think it is better for me to weigh myself twice a week for now, because I wasn't lying in bed worrying about what it was going to say. Have a great day. I know I will, and no, I am not going to celebrate the weight loss with a milk shake. It is motivating to stay on track! THANK YOU!!!"

Suzanne's Journal Notes …

"I wore my new black blouse tucked into my grey dress slacks—yes, I said tucked in! Today was the first day I really felt thinner. I know the positive weight loss was part of it, but I haven't tucked in a blouse in a long time, and there was still room in my pants."

What a great feeling, being able to tuck in her shirt.

Sunday, March 11

Suzanne's Journal Notes…

"We have a major kitchen problem. There is a leak under the sink and dishwasher that we think has been going on for a while. It has ruined the cabinet and the insulation in the basement. The flooring is all warped, so…we have the plumber coming tomorrow and have to call in Joe. The problem is we can't use the sink, etc. and no cooking."

Monday, March 12

Suzanne's Journal Notes …

"It's a beautiful day today. It is going up close to 60 and the sun is shining. I decided to wear a new blouse and I

have already gotten at least five compliments today—one from a stranger I passed in the office building. So, is it the blouse, my posture, do I just look better? Whatever it is, it is certainly making me feel good."

Compliments—especially compliments from strangers—will keep Suzanne motivated.

Tuesday, March 13

I noticed how great Suzanne looked as soon as she walked into the WRN luncheon. We sat next to each other and she told me how supportive Kris is getting of her exercise routine. He's believing her and seeing her commitment to getting fit. "It's not impacting Kris" and this is part of the reason for his being supportive of her program. Suzanne is changing her life and people will wonder what impact it will have on their relationship with her. For Kris, there's no negative impact, only positive.

Thursday, March 15

I arrived at Suzanne's house at 8:00 a.m. and she greeted me in their gorgeous kitchen. Tucker the dog and Ian the almost-7-year-old were there, too.

As I was coming out of their incredibly decorated bathroom, Suzanne was putting in a load of wash. She does about twelve loads a week. She said sometimes the boys wear something for an hour or pick it out of a drawer and don't want to wear it or fold it, so it gets thrown in the laundry. Whoops, we did it when we were younger—sorry Mom!

Last evening Kris told Suzanne he is having someone over for dinner tonight so she was scurrying around to create a menu.

We went to the basement with Tucker leading the way and Ian taking up the rear. Ian has quite a lot of Lego building blocks spread on the floor, but they had been moved away from Suzanne's workout area.

I sat in the "comfortable chair" because Tucker likes to lie on the sofa behind Suzanne. "I did cheat." Oh, what would Suzanne say next? "I got on the scale. 145 pounds. I jumped up and down a few times and it was 145." She's reached her new goal weight mid-March!

Is she eating the chocolates at work? "No, but it was hard." We talked about making sure she answered her chocolate craving. "Yes, there has to be chocolate."

Is she feeling deprived? "No!" Suzanne is learning to listen to her body by eating the foods she enjoys—even chocolate—in moderation.

I asked if she still likes food. "Oh gosh, I love food!"

Suzanne shared a milestone she had reached. Recently there were 15 people at her sister Karen's house and Suzanne was standing in front of the food, picking at the appetizers. Suzanne realized she didn't want to pick at the food, so she went into the kitchen to help her sister cook the meal—just the two of them. Suzanne and Karen don't always get to spend time together, so this was a special time for them. Several days later Suzanne received an email from her sister saying how much fun she had had with Suzanne. When Suzanne and I first started working together, she was fixated more on the food than on the people. Karen's email is living proof that Suzanne is slowly changing her thinking. Suzanne's journey is having a positive impact on her relationship with Karen.

"I was 145 this morning! Could I be in the 130s?"

Friday, March 16

Suzanne's Journal Notes...

"Last night I woke up about 1:30 a.m. with a bad case of GERD (Gastro Esophageal Reflux Disease). I don't know what that is about. That's the second time in about a month I have had an attack, and before that it had been a year. I still don't feel really well today. My stomach just kind of feels sour. I think I'll call the doctor this afternoon to see if there is something I should have on hand for these episodes. Not fun!"

I'm not a doctor, but if she's eating a large meal then exercising two hours later, she should keep an eye on it. Suzanne's doctor recommended taking an over-the-counter drug.

Sunday, March 18

Suzanne's Journal Notes ...

"I slept okay last night—thank goodness. It's the third day of the medicine and the GERD is still acting up. I have never had the GERD constantly like this. Definitely not feeling like exercise tonight. 8:45 p.m., I did only 15 minutes on the step and I took it a little slow. I did the push-ups and abs. I hope I sleep tonight!"

Suzanne is listening to her body by cutting way back on her exercises.

Monday, March 19

An email came in from Suzanne:

"Hi Linda, What is the plan for our workout tomorrow, inside or outside? How much space do we need? I am just trying to figure out if we are working out in the house, what I need to clean up to have room for us. See you tomorrow morning."

I wrote back that we'd need space inside and will surprise her with kick boxing.

Tuesday, March 20

I arrived early at Suzanne's house and she was standing at the bus stop chatting with a neighbor. Suzanne said to come in now, even though she hadn't cleaned off the counters. She does like a neat house.

Suzanne was still not feeling well. We (Tucker, Suzanne and I) went to the basement and she elaborated on that feeling. It hurts under her bra line and behind her back, so I'm glad she contacted her doctor. The GERD is coming at night. Jokingly I asked if it was her body responding to this weight loss and exercise. Suzanne answered that it was her body responding to no chocolate. Actually, she knows not to deprive herself of chocolate and was proud to report that she had bought a bag, unopened since last Thursday.

She looks slim and has long, lean legs. The pants Suzanne wanted to wear were in the wash so she put on yoga pants. She remarked that she has a lot of work to do on her legs and commented about her stomach while grabbing it. I explained that what she was grabbing was about five pounds of fatty tissue. "Really?"

We went back to the GERD. Her mom suffers from it too, but I don't know if this is hereditary. Because of GERD, her mom has given up certain things, which Suzanne might have to do, too. We need to keep an eye on it and I told her it started when she increased the intensity of the step. "I don't like the possible solution," Suzanne said. My thought is—and I'm not a doctor—for her to cut back on the intensity of her step routine when she's had a big meal. Her current schedule is 6:30 p.m. dinner, 8:30 p.m. step then 10:30 p.m. bed. She talked about stepping at 6:00 p.m. but isn't sure. Suzanne needs to fit in the exercise whenever she can. I don't want her taking medicine so she can exercise—that doesn't make sense. And if the exercise intensity is too high so close to a meal and bed, she has to listen to her body and cut back. Suzanne's concern is that she wants to do some form of cardio so we need to find something that agrees with her system. She talked about walking as fast as she could with KJ, but how she sweats when she does step. Her current eating and exercise pattern cannot continue if she has to take medication to do it.

Suzanne is looking forward to her trip to Puerto Rico. She told me, "While I'm away I have no agenda so I get to solve the world's problems. I've never ever done this before—I'm packing my sneakers. The hotel has a gym so I might attempt to try the equipment while not embarrassing myself."

Suzanne is constantly in motion—both her body and brain—so we talked about meditation. She needs to take time to relax and it could be something as simple as taking time to read a magazine. This means no creating a shopping list, no Mom's taxi, nothing like that; just relax.

Suzanne told me that she was looking at a magazine the other day and noticed there was a 20-minute workout in it. Before, she would have read the magazine, gotten to the workout section and said, "Oh, that's nice," then continued reading. Now, she might try the workout. She pointed out that the magazine workout included the plank. "I do the plank," she said, oozing with confidence.

Number Two on my checklist was a plan for Puerto Rico, but Suzanne already had this covered. Historically, a buffet is not a good thing, but she has a plan to have a vegetable omelet and fresh fruit. She said they might have a later breakfast, a light lunch then dinner.

"The thing that bugs me is that I'll spend a fortune on water. I just have to get over it. Still, I do have to mentally prepare."

She talked about needing new sneakers and hopes to get them before they go away.

"I'm nervous about us working out together." In the past I've given Suzanne exercises and she's done them on her own. Now, she's working out with me. She hasn't taken formal classes in six years so kick boxing was something new to her. Lesson learned—she had on the wrong sports bra and it didn't give her enough support.

Suzanne knew most of the songs on my "Soul Music" CD and I could tell she was getting into the music. This is why she missed taking classes—music and working out with others, in this case, me. She kept saying how much she loved what we were doing. We boxed for 20 minutes and she had enough energy to sing part of a song. We were both sweaty and she was able to regulate her breathing the entire time. "Woo, I love it!"

When I got home I emailed Suzanne that in the next day or two she might be a little sore. Sometimes muscle soreness isn't felt till 24-48 hours after the activity. If she feels anything, she's to let me know when and where. For music, I asked if she likes 80s or disco. To help her justify purchasing water in Puerto Rico, I wrote that all the money she saved on not purchasing exercise equipment or a gym membership could be spent on water.

Her reply:

> *"You're the best!! Thanks for the workout. I loved it. And it did make me realize how much I enjoyed going to a class and also how much difference the music makes! I love either 80s or disco. And you are so right about the water."*

Suzanne likes to journal while she's on vacation, so she'll do so in Puerto Rico. I suggested she write more detail about GERD; something is triggering it. Going on vacation is a great time to try new things, so it's okay if she doesn't get in all of her exercises or water. Suzanne mentioned that she might try to exercise in the morning. I'm eager to see how Suzanne's GERD responds to her exercising earlier instead of later in the day or evening like she has been.

Suzanne's Journal Notes ...

> *"Since I worked out with Linda in the morning, I did not step tonight. I had a meeting for KJ's tennis at 7:00 p.m. and didn't get home until almost 9:00 p.m. After I read to Ian and he went to bed, I decided to just completely chill out and I chose not to do the abs and push-ups at that hour to see how my body reacts. I still took two antacids before bed, but I slept okay."*

This is the first time since January that Suzanne has not done her daily exercises. She listened to her body.

Wednesday, March 21

Suzanne's Journal Notes ...

> *"Like Linda and I were talking yesterday—do you have to be miserable or unhappy to be stressed? I am certainly not unhappy or miserable. But life is very full right now.*

> *"And tonight will be another night where I keep going until after KJ gets finished with a tutoring session about 8:00 p.m. I do, however, have a wonderful lunch planned with girlfriends today and I am getting my hair done this afternoon. So I will have some time to relax. I am still taking the medicine for GERD."*

I sent Suzanne an email saying she's been stepping close to when she's consumed a meal. Would she like to try something totally different? Instead of stepping, how about she use that time to take a bubble bath, read or do something relaxing so her brain doesn't have to think and her body doesn't have to function at an intense step workout level. She could still walk, ride her bike and do her exercises whenever she wanted, just not within a few hours of consuming a big meal. If Suzanne chooses to do this, I will be very eager to see what happens to her body.

> *"Hi Linda, I am afraid of two things: (1) once I sit and relax, I am afraid I won't get back up and (2) if not then, when to exercise? I had lunch today with Carol and Caitlin. Remember—they are my skinny fitness friends. Caitlin suggested I try the 5:30-5:45 a.m. time. She says it's hard to get up, but once you're up and get your workout in, it's done for the day. It really did feel good to have exercised with you yesterday morning. I am going to do a 15-minute step tonight, maybe not quite as intense. I am feeling better today, and I didn't eat a very big dinner, but I don't want to push it. We'll see what tomorrow brings, but maybe I'll try the early thing tomorrow or Friday. Thanks again!"*

Thursday, March 22

I leave today to visit my parents in Florida. It will be strange not having email contact with Suzanne until Tuesday. I gave her my cell number just in case she needs to call. She's going through some serious changes in her life and it's important that she know I'm just a phone call away.

Tuesday, March 27

I received an email:

> "Hi Linda and welcome home! I hope you had a great
> and relaxing trip. I am busy getting ready for our vacation
> and Kris is out of town again. I know we are meeting
> tomorrow. What did you have planned? I am a little
> concerned about the sweating thing. I will have to go
> back to work, so I'll have to be able to re-dress or stay
> dressed for work. Or should we meet for lunch? If you
> get a chance to let me know before our meeting great,
> otherwise I'll plan to meet you at my house at 11:00 a.m.
> I will do my best to remember to email you my journal in
> the morning. See you tomorrow."

Wednesday, March 28

Instead of working out, Suzanne and I met for lunch. We hugged hi and I thought to myself that she really does look good! I swear people have a different air about them when they gain control of their lives. She looked cute wearing her new white sneakers. She looked confident. She looked happy, really happy!

Suzanne told me about the two families that came unexpectedly to her home last Saturday evening. She worked till 5:00 p.m., stopped at the grocery store then came home to cook. I always take notes when we meet, so she said, "Write down in bold lettering, 'Suzanne threw out a slew of stuff.'"

Suzanne shocked me when she said she had stepped already this morning. Since she didn't work out Saturday, she worked out twice on Sunday. I think missing Saturday's cardio workout is the first time in a long time for her.

She told me she's looking forward to eating chocolate at the end of the month. One of Suzanne's goals was to not eat chocolate at work because she considered it mindless eating.

I was looking at the big white fried chips on the table in the Chinese restaurant when Suzanne said, "They're bad for you." Speaking of bad, I told her I had a donut this morning. She looked shocked and surprised, but I wanted her to know personal trainers are human. The difference is, I only ate one and the last time I had a donut was about a month ago.

Since I have an intense tennis clinic after our meeting, I asked if Suzanne minded if I ordered just soup. "I'm getting over it, sort of." Poor Suzanne. For her, I take all the fun out of eating. I ordered soup and she got a sushi box.

Suzanne has been taking GERD medicine for two weeks and said, "My stomach is fine!" She will remember that a big dinner and heart-pumping cardio are not a good combination. Last Thursday she started exercising in the morning and it's agreeing with her body, the inside of her body.

"The highlight of Sunday was bicycling with my little one." Ian got a bike last Christmas and wasn't too interested in it. He even told his parents he didn't need it. The other day KJ rode it and suddenly Ian liked his new bike. To have Ian and Suzanne out there riding for a half hour and for her to say it was the highlight of her Sunday—this is something money can't buy. Suzanne is accomplishing several goals: make exercise fun and work out with the kids.

Suzanne left her To Do list at the mall so she is going back to pick it up. She wants to cross off what she had done. She's so busy getting ready for vacation, yet she is going to take 20 minutes out of her day to go back to the mall. The main reason was that she had taken the time to generate the list and empty her head of it. She didn't want to take the time to re-create the list and then wonder if she had forgotten to put something back on it. Is part of Suzanne's success this desire to accomplish what is on her list?

I asked if she had tried on her bathing suits and we even talked about a bikini. "I might wear a bikini," she said cautiously.

Did she feel okay after kick boxing? "Oh yeah, I loved that! And I was a little bit sore up here (shoulders). I tried doing kick boxing on my own and it wasn't fun."

As people notice Suzanne's weight loss, they ask her what she is doing. She asked me, "What am I on?" She's not on anything, especially not a diet.

"One evening Kris said there's a whole different aura about me." Wow, talk about a motivating statement.

Suzanne said she envisions a lifestyle of getting up in the morning to exercise on Monday, Wednesday and Friday, constant exercise. She doesn't want to yo-yo her weight and wants to be in maintenance mode. "Long-term, I want healthy living."

We talked about Kris, his job, their family, his family and their dinner Friday evening. All of these things are important to her. If an issue is happening in Suzanne's household and it's hindering her from exercising, she has to learn to deal with the issue. She can't go around a problem; she has to go through it.

While we were eating Suzanne kept talking about the delicious almond cookie they will give us with our check. When the waiter brought us fortune cookies she said, "What, no almond cookies?" Apparently almond cookies only come with dinner, but he brought us some. The cookies were so-so tasting and Suzanne explained that she had been hungrier last week, so the cookie was tastier then. Suzanne smiled when I read my fortune: "You will be successful in your work." I told her my success is sitting right across the table from me. Suzanne wanted to save her fortune cookie for her afternoon snack.

Friday, March 30

Suzanne's Journal Notes ...

"I met my weight goal with two pounds to spare! We're on our way to Puerto Rico. We got up at 5:00 a.m. in order to make our flight. It was really hard leaving KJ behind (he was staying with friends because of his sports

schedule), especially since the other kids are so excited. I know we're going to have a great time and so will KJ. He has tons of tennis to play and he'll enjoy being with his cousins. Every time I vacation, I really enjoy the time to just clear my mind and allow myself to think about our life and dream and plan and organize. I always come home thinking I can do anything. This is the first time that I have gone on a vacation and intentionally packed my sneakers and special clothes for exercising. Even my exercise bands are packed! I am really in a good place—13 lbs. thinner than Christmas. I haven't had my bathing suit on yet and even though I probably won't be satisfied, I already know I will look better than I did last August! And trying on some of my summer clothes last night was very rewarding—they fit well!"

Saturday, March 31

Suzanne's Journal Notes ...

"Well, life is tough. I'm updating my journal poolside at the El San Juan. I was just spritzed by the pool girls. It's a beautiful sunny day with a great breeze. The pool area is hopping. It's Saturday, so I'm assuming it's the busiest day. This morning I went to the gym with Griffin. We made a pact to go together every day. I did 1.5 miles on the elliptical machine. It took 17 minutes and I averaged about 6 mph. Okay, so nobody else would be impressed, but I was impressed with myself. I haven't been in a gym for about six years. It was loaded with machines, mirrors and obviously fit people. But I put on my workout clothes and joined them—a big step for me. I also did my old five-pound weight routine for my arms, although they felt like 10-pound weights. I did 20 push-ups and the abs routine—eight planks, 12 push-ups, 20 four-count sit-ups, 12 side abs and 20 reverse curls sit-ups. Then Grif and I

met up with Kris and Ian poolside. We went to a coffee place for breakfast at around 10:00 a.m. I had a nonfat mocha, yogurt (60 calories) and a slice of banana nut bread. Oh, and with the workout, 20 ounces of water.

"1:00 p.m., frozen drink poolside—absolute heaven! We just ordered lunch and I ordered a fruit boat—what is happening to me? It's all good. The fruit boat came—way too little fruit and four big slices of banana nut bread. I ate 1½ pieces of the banana nut bread and all of the fruit. Later, I went for a great walk on the beach. I kept it brisk, but no watch, so I don't know how long I walked. Ian started to lose it and he hadn't eaten anything healthy, so we went and got him an order of chicken fingers and me a garden salad and went back to the room. It was the best plan. The chicken fingers were really good and then I really didn't care what he ate for dinner. We chilled out to "Father of the Bride" and it really rejuvenated him for the evening. The salad and a roll was just what I was craving. We ate dinner at about 7:30 at the Ranch restaurant. I had a frozen margarita, some nachos and baby back ribs. I left about six ribs and I had some coleslaw, too—and more water. After dinner the kids had gelato. We hung out in the lobby for a little while, then the kids went to bed and Kris & I checked out the casino. I couldn't stay. I really enjoy watching other people play, but not Kris. I don't like the idea of losing money, but Kris really enjoys playing. I was happy flipping between the basketball game and ice skating."

March was a wonderful month for Suzanne. Her husband noticed a difference in her. She exercised with her son. She tucked in her shirt. She got a compliment from a stranger. She spent time in the kitchen with her sister. GERD was dealt with and we think we figured out what was causing it. We exercised together. And, for their Puerto Rico vacation, she packed her workout clothes and actually worked out in the hotel gym.

To Do:

1. Be aware of what you are eating

2. Continue to set monthly goals

3. Keep changing up your monthly exercise routine

4. Let the weather dictate your activity

5. When your body talks to you, listen to it

April:

Stalled at a New Size

Sunday, April 1

Suzanne's Journal Notes...

"A gorgeous day in Puerto Rico; hotter today than the other days! 8:15 a.m. Griffin and I were at the gym. I did 25 minutes on the elliptical machine (including five minutes of cool-down. I did the arms with the weights again, 20 push-ups and some abs. I feel like a million bucks.

"9:30 a.m. another breakfast at the coffee place. I had the 60-calorie yogurt and fruit and a non-fat, no-whip mocha. After breakfast I bought a new bikini. I am poolside with my wrinkled stomach hanging out. I see a little bit of everything down here. OK, there are definitely some beautifully built women, but there are even more women that don't have beautiful bodies, but they walk with a certain confidence that I really admire."

How exciting that Suzanne bought a bikini. I hope she gains the confidence to wear it this summer...I think she will.

Monday, April 2

Suzanne's Journal Notes...

"8:15 a.m. workout at the gym. I used the Cybex machine today. It was kind of like a cross between the elliptical and a step machine. I did 20 minutes and burned 185 calories. We did arms, push-ups and abs like the other days. Another great workout made even better by Griffin's company. It started out raining this morning, but

quickly improved. We walked to a different restaurant for breakfast. I ate half of my omelet. It was horrible and the service even worse. I also had half an English muffin with a little butter, small OJ and a cup of coffee with cream and Sweet'N Low. I also had a few bites of the boys' pancakes. For lunch (about 2:00 p.m.) we had a pizza and chicken fingers. I ate two pieces of pizza and two bites of chicken fingers. We had water all day and then one frozen drink. We still haven't decided on dinner yet, but another great day at the beach and pool."

On vacation Kris sleeps in, so Suzanne used to hang around till he got up. This time she took advantage of the time by going to the gym. One of her goals was to make exercise fun and another was to incorporate her kids. She's accomplished two of her goals.

Tuesday, April 3

Suzanne's Journal Notes ...

"It's not even 8:00 a.m. and I came down to the pool and literally got the last two chairs. Thankfully, I brought an extra magazine to leave here and save the spot. The only problem, this spot is in the front row and there is no way to hide in my bikini. I am feeling really bloated today. I don't know why. I feel like I've eaten pretty well—maybe I still need more water. I am here at the pool just waiting for Griffin to go to the gym. It looks like it's going to be a beautiful day.

"After our workout, we ended our day early at the pool and went by taxi to the El Morro fort and then tee-shirt shopping in Old San Juan. We had my favorite meal of the vacation at the Parrot Club in Old San Juan. I had their signature frozen fruity cocktail, followed by lots of water. We had ceviche and different grilled meats for appetizers. For dinner I had the steak churrasco (like a

skirt steak), with a stuffed pepper and something made out of corn. I almost completely finished my plate it was all so delicious!"

Wednesday, April 4

Suzanne's Journal Notes ...

"8:30 a.m. workout at the gym. I used the elliptical machine today for 20 minutes plus the four-minute cooldown. I burned about 200 calories and went about two miles. I did my same arms, push-ups and abs. We had breakfast at the coffee shop once again. They only had the high-test yogurt, which was 150 calories, but it was really good. I had the yogurt, fruit and mocha again. Today is our day to go home, so we only spent a couple hours at the pool.

"At 1:00 we arrived at the airport. While the plane was still loading, the flight attendant came up to Kris and said they had a family that needed to sit together and would we mind moving to business class. Would we mind—are you crazy? Send me up!!! Now, why they just didn't put the other family up there I cannot explain, but I was just grateful. We hardly were seated when they asked us what we would like to drink. I already had water, so I didn't have anything. But we had a choice of meals. I had the salad with grilled chicken and fat-free vinaigrette with a roll with a little butter. And I had one bite of Griffin's cheesecake. And then we were home and reality of work, etc. all came flying back almost as quickly as I set it aside!"

Suzanne was on vacation yet she worked out each morning. She didn't mention GERD, which might mean working out in the morning agreed with her system.

Thursday, April 5

> *"Good Morning Linda, We got home around 10:00 last night. I did not get my picture taken this morning—all of my workout clothes were still dirty and in the suitcase, so I will definitely get it done tomorrow morning. I also have not typed my journal into the computer yet. I will hopefully get that done tonight and send it to you tomorrow. The great news is (1) I worked out in the hotel gym every day and it was awesome and (2) I weighed 144 this morning. I wasn't going to get on the scale today, but I thought why not...more later. Suz"*

Suzanne was concerned about gaining weight on vacation so I asked if she was going to Puerto Rico to eat or to enjoy the scenery and her family. She maintained her weight because she didn't eat much, drank lots of water, exercised and kept a journal. There was no magic pill; it was a combination of these four things. She is slowly learning that life is not about food and she is slowly detaching from it. Life can revolve around food but food is not the answer.

When people learn Suzanne and I are working together, they say I must be proud of what I did for Suzanne. My response is that I am proud of Suzanne for what she did. I didn't go on vacation with her but mentally she had me there. I'm not with her every day but she knows I'm a phone call or email away. This journey is all about her.

As I write this, I still struggle to find the solution to her journey, if there is one, to help those who don't get it. Is it about timing? I feel that timing is critical, because if Suzanne and I had worked together a year ago, she might not have had the same results. And I feel it has a lot to do with personality. Some clients will always struggle while others will embrace what I share with them and make it work for them.

There are so many exciting things about Suzanne, but a main one is watching her gain self-confidence. She has a new air about her and she's different—she has a different outlook on life. She's happy. She's fun to be around. She enjoys life.

Friday, April 6

Suzanne's Journal Notes ...

"It was picture day, and then I wore my picture clothes to work out. Two months ago, I wouldn't have left my bedroom in that outfit!"

Monday, April 9

I arrived at Suzanne's house just before 8:00 a.m. and knocked quietly because the kids were home for spring break. Suzanne answered the door in a hooded sweatshirt, new white sneaks and shorts with Puerto Rico-tanned legs. She has great legs!

We went right into the basement and she handed me her pictures. "Ugh, I don't think they're too good. I feel the weight loss, though." We compared previous pictures and we could see a difference in the pictures of her back.

When I commented about her bikini she said, "I did it!" Suzanne doesn't like her stomach, yet she was on vacation wearing a two-piece. Wow!

She put her foot down yesterday with a situation that happened at home. Prior to our working together, Suzanne might not have been so forceful with her feelings. She might have said, "Okay," but it wouldn't have been okay. Part of what Suzanne is doing is building a strong body and the other part, the more important part, is building a strong mind. As she feels in control of her body, she gains confidence. Now, Suzanne puts up with less, commands respect, speaks up and tells people how she feels.

"Easter Sunday was not a good eating day. I told myself to get my butt on the scale this morning. It was not quite 145 and not quite 144. I had thought it might be 146 pounds."

Ian, who informed me he will turn seven on Thursday, and Tucker were downstairs with us. Ian had to show me a new Lego truck he had gotten that has 1,000 pieces. Suzanne just had him pick up the train set off the floor and now he's going to start a huge Lego truck project.

She rearranged the chairs to give us more room to work out and she is starting to take charge of her workout space.

I asked if there was anything else she wanted to discuss before we started working out. "I'm waiting for you to ask me the question. I've been thinking about it for three days." Darn, I wasn't sure what Suzanne was talking about so I went over my checklist. The only other thing to discuss was her April goals, so I said that out loud. "Yes! I've been thinking about goals for three days and this is what I came up with: 140, but I'm really, really nervous about it. I'm already scared. Instead of by the end of April, should it be by the end of May or the end of the year? My exercise goal sounds simple but I'd like to move the cardio to 20 minutes, five times a week. My food goal, instead of avoiding chocolates in the work bowl, is to eat fruit each day. Is that okay? I have to write these down." Her goals were right on target and I liked her creativity. Since she's doing fine with drinking water, we're not going to touch that goal; we'll leave it as it is.

Suzanne talked about constipation. With the changes in her food and liquid intake she can very well experience constipation or diarrhea. I told her about high fiber cereals and in particular Fiber One. She can put Fiber One in a cup of yogurt or eat it like cereal, with milk. I cautioned her because a serving contains 13 grams of fiber, versus her other breakfast cereal, which might have six grams or less. She has to slowly build up her intake of fiber so she doesn't have repercussions. For fruit, she's to pick something with a skin on it like an apple or pear or other fruits she likes. The combination of fiber cereal, water and fruit will help clean out her colon and give her a more regular bowel movement.

Ian was intrigued with the new stability ball I had brought Suzanne and wanted to play with it but Suzanne said no. He also wanted to open up his 1,000-piece Lego truck kit and tried several times, but Suzanne said no. She stuck to what she said and followed through with Ian; 'no' meant 'no'. Is this a character trait that has helped her lose weight and be disciplined?

Suzanne took off her hooded sweatshirt and she had on a new white sleeveless shirt, which she bought when she got her sneaks. She is showing off a lot of skin, which is a great indicator that she is feeling more comfortable in her own skin (a goal she originally told me when we first met).

Ian asked if I was going to stay all day and I said yes, because I want his mom to cook for me. Suzanne said, "I would cook for you, but you probably wouldn't eat anything and then I'd feel like you didn't like it."

Suzanne asked Ian how she looked in her bikini. "Pretty nice!" Children can be brutally honest and will tell the truth, whether we want to hear it or not. In this case, we wanted to hear it.

We went over the new ball routine and Suzanne will do this routine daily along with her cardio workout.

I said I wanted a picture of her in the bikini. "Oh, I don't know."

I left around 9:30 a.m. and started thinking about her personality traits. She doesn't like confrontation, so she likes to please people, or better yet, she likes to keep the peace. She followed through with Ian—'no' meant 'no'—and she was firm about that. Are these two more personality traits that have helped her to be so successful?

I definitely want Suzanne to come to work with me as a trainer. She's been on this journey and she knows how it feels. I'm willing to wait years for her because she's worth it. And I might start taking Suzanne with me when I do presentations. I've done this before—brought a client with me. It is one thing for the audience to hear about weight loss and lifestyle changes, but it's another thing to see the person. She's living proof that what we're doing works.

Suzanne told me I make all things seem possible. It's true because I break down the task into manageable pieces and make sure she's taking small steps toward her goals. Realistic expectations have been set so she can succeed, which continues to motivate her.

Suzanne's Journal Notes ...

"Dinner: 7:00 p.m. I made a new recipe. We had frisee and baby spinach salad, garlic shrimp and spaghetti with peas and zucchini ribbons and blackberry crumble for dessert. The spaghetti was tossed with yogurt. I can't find the nutrition information to get the calorie count, but I don't think it was too bad. There wasn't a lot of sugar added to the blackberries and I figure it counts toward my fruit intake. ☺ 16 ounces of water."

Tuesday, April 10

I was early to the Women's Referral Network luncheon and was already in the room when I noticed Suzanne. She was stunning and created a presence. She was tanned and wore a gray sweater, white shirt, unique silver necklace, tight black pants, big belt and boots with a heel. She has the longest legs and they are very lean. When I commented on her belt buckle, she pointed to her shirt and said, "It's tucked in. I figured 'why not?'" When a woman who normally doesn't tuck in a shirt tucks it in, it's monumental.

We bumped into another client—Katherine—who had lost 40 pounds. She and Suzanne had fun chatting about what they had done to lose their weight. Both said the same things: keep a journal, drink water, exercise.

During the luncheon we went around the table telling how we promote women's health in our business. This was an easy question for me to answer. I told the eight women at my table that Suzanne tucked in her shirt. Some nodded their heads with envy. I said tucking in a shirt might not seem like a big deal for some people, but it is. A woman who had her shirt out said that it is a big deal.

After the luncheon I had a wild idea to have someone take a picture of us—me, Katherine and Suzanne. It's not often that I see clients dressed up—they're always in workout clothes.

I saw the old Suzanne today—the one who was the president of the WRN, the one who seemed to have all her ducks in a row and the one whom I wanted to emulate as a business person. She is reemerging as a very confident woman. And it's only going to get better. When she gets down to 140 and into the 130s, she's going to be unstoppable. It's not about the weight; it's about the confidence. The sky will be the limit and her opportunities will be endless.

Thursday, April 12

Suzanne's Journal Notes ...

"What a day I had! I know it's all in the planning, and planning I did. Today was Ian's birthday, and unfortunately with the schedule we've been keeping, I had not put a fair amount of effort in before today. So the day started at 5:45 a.m. when I rose to do my exercises—yea to checking that off the list. We got ready (Ian showered, too) and left in time to pick up soft pretzels to take to his class to celebrate his birthday, drop off a tax return and get him to school by 8:50 a.m. Then to the office, work, work, work, and then I left at 11:15 a.m. to go back to school to do my Instructional Support in Ian's classroom. I had a quick lunch at home before heading to see a client to do their monthly accounting work until 4:30 p.m. At 4:30 p.m. it was off to Target for party plates and napkins, to Giant for the ever-so-delicious Hamburger Helper ingredients (and a HB balloon), into the Exton Mall to pick up the birthday cookie and a stop at the karate school to pick up his uniform. I got home in time to make dinner for us (including mom, and a fresh salad for those of us who should not be living on Hamburger Helper alone), eat, open presents, sing Happy Birthday and do two tax returns until 10:15 p.m. I did my exercises and crashed."

Talk about dedication. After a long and exhausting day like this, Suzanne still did her exercises.

Friday, April 13

Suzanne's Journal Notes ...

"144 lbs. – Well, the weight certainly had me depressed this morning. And needless to say, I am feeling a little sluggish. I guess that makes sense after my day yesterday. Yesterday I felt pretty empowered because I actually got everything done I had to get done. I still have a few client headaches to deal with today that kind of have me frustrated. I guess I am at another one of those stuck spots where it's up to me to take the next leap in order to drop some more weight. I guess I am kind of bummed about it because we have a dinner out with friends tonight and I know it will be really hard to eat sensibly. We also have my family all coming to celebrate Ian's birthday tomorrow night and we're having pizza and more dessert. Sunday I have a shower to go to.

"Now, while I was stepping this morning I was trying to get myself out of this funky mood. I am trying to convince myself that it is not just about the weight and I have successfully gotten through vacation, Easter, tax season and one birthday without gaining any weight. I should be really pleased. I know I look better in my clothes and that was one of the main goals. Maybe it's just the day, and I have to get the work out of the way, or the hormones are not aligned right—who knows, but I have to keep going. And right now I have to get going to the shower or the rest of the day I'll be trying to catch up!"

I sent Suzanne an email. Initially this journey wasn't about weight, but her April goal of 140 pounds has put some pressure on her. To help, I suggested bumping up her water intake each day. I told her that when she goes to all these social functions over the weekend, she should enjoy the food in moderation and focus on the social part. I agree that she should be really pleased because she feels better, looks better in her clothes, tucked in her shirt, wore a bikini on vacation and maintained her weight through vacation, Easter, tax season and a birthday.

Sunday, April 15

Suzanne's Journal Notes …

"It was a nor'easter storm this morning and I was really enjoying lying in bed and listening to the rain, but I decided to push through and I got up and did 20+ minutes of step, took a quick shower and made it to church. KJ decided to come with me, which of course was wonderful. After church we picked up bagels. I had a sesame bagel with lettuce, tomato, cucumbers, pine nut spread and veggie schmear. It was really good (that was about 11:30 a.m.).

"We had Kandi's shower today and thankfully, Kris decided that he'd drive me up to the shower and the boys could spend the afternoon together. There were a lot of great snacks and I probably ate too many. I had veggies and lots of pineapple and cantaloupe. I had bruschetta with fresh mozzarella, spinach dip with rye bread, chicken salad with flat bread and three crackers with baked cream cheese. I had a piece of cake and iced tea. All these snacks were between 2:30 and 5:00 p.m. I didn't eat after that except for four spoonfuls of leftover Hamburger Helper and at least 40 ounces of water."

Why do we serve so many unhealthful things at parties, showers and other special occasions? Women attend many of these functions, they're trying to lose weight or at least watch what they eat, yet we continue to serve these items. Sometimes I think it's an excuse to serve and eat junk food. Considering her options, Suzanne made healthy choices.

Tuesday, April 17

I received an email from Suzanne with "Howdy!" in the subject line:

> *"Well, I've officially made it through tax season; I'm not quite finished with my own returns yet, but pretty soon. I was 143 pounds this morning; the pressure is on. Just a thought in advance of our meeting on Thursday...do you have one or two additional abs exercises for the ball? I am not feeling like I am getting quite enough abs work in the new routine. For some reason the reverse curls seem easy; maybe I'm doing something wrong. I tried lifting my head and it still seems pretty easy. I put the ball along with the step in the car on Thursday. Thank you!"*

Suzanne is asking for more abs exercises? She's not feeling the reverse curl? The reverse curl is the one she had trouble doing. That is serious progress.

Thursday, April 19

Suzanne looked adorable in her new workout outfit. It was a matching blue jacket and crop pants along with her new white sneakers and new white sleeveless shirt. She was 144.5 pounds the last time I saw her and as of Tuesday, she was 143 pounds.

We ran through her April goals: weight is 143 pounds, she's doing at least five days of a 20-minute cardio workout and she's eating fruit daily.

Suzanne shared a story with me: The family was going out to an Italian restaurant but ended up at a burger shop, even though Suzanne voted against it. A milestone happened—instead of ordering a cheeseburger she had her first veggie burger.

Suzanne is proud of her weight loss and is telling people about it. We talked about where the 14 pounds were coming off. "My boobs are smaller. I like having them out of the way. Bras are smaller, better." Suzanne said her "little success" was warming up using the first step routine then doing the second step routine. She's mixing things up on her own and seeing and feeling progress.

Suzanne was trying to read her notes and do a new step routine. Did she want the music on? "Yes, because I like it." When she got to the Fast Feet, "I'm not graceful at these. And, yes, my heart rate is up. You can hear it."

As we were cooling down, it was the perfect time to ask Suzanne if she wanted to work together through June. Our conversation about this lasted a lot longer than I had expected. Did she want to? "Yes!" But she seemed puzzled. "Am I doing okay?" She was doing fine but I have more things I want to accomplish with her and I need June to do them.

"My goals from our first meeting at the Chinese restaurant aren't good enough." Goals change because she's achieved all that she wanted to. "I never would have 143 pounds as a goal because I didn't think it was possible. Now, 135 pounds swirls in my mind. Am I doing okay?" I reassured her that she was doing an unbelievable job. I couldn't ask for more.

Suzanne is used to doing her nightly exercises upstairs but now there's a logistic challenge; the stability ball is in the basement. She has to create a new pattern and I'm hoping it won't be too much of an issue. Convenience is important and the ball being in the basement is not convenient.

Today for the first time, I saw Suzanne's stomach. She always comments about it being wrinkly, so I said she has two choices: learn to deal with it or get plastic surgery. She said no one sees it but she does look at other people's stomachs. What Suzanne doesn't realize is that some women would kill for her body—even her wrinkly stomach.

I got a long hug goodbye and she said, "You're the best!" The compliment was greatly appreciated but I struggle with how to help other clients be and feel as successful as Suzanne.

Tuesday, April 24

Suzanne's Journal Notes ...

"6:00 a.m. 25 minutes of step. I weighed myself as soon as I got up and I was somewhere between 143 and 144 pounds. I felt as if I deserved that weight because I felt

like I was doing nonsense eating yesterday. The pretzel sandwiches, the two pretzel nuggets and the ice cream could and should have been avoided, but I still munched. After I finished the step today I got back on the scale and weighed 142. I guess that probably was cheating, but it at least temporarily made me feel better. Actually, just the workout made me feel better.

"Dinner: 6:30 p.m., shrimp Caesar. The magazine menu called for breadsticks to go with the salad. I ate the serving size they suggested and later looked up the calories. I think I added almost 400 calories to my healthy salad. Why would the magazine do that? Maybe I am off with my calorie count, but it was like eating two pieces of bread. I knew it must have been too good to be true! I also had 16 ounces of water."

Her breadsticks comment reminds me of a baked potato—low in calories till you top it with butter, sour cream, bacon bits and cheese.

Wednesday, April 25

When I arrived at the coffee shop Suzanne was already there. She got up and gave me a big hug; she seems so happy. Since I'm not a coffee person and didn't know what to get, I ordered what she did…a tall, nonfat, no-whip mocha. "We're getting some chocolate with the mocha."

"It's not a good weight week. My weight is playing games." Suzanne has lost 14 pounds since January and needs to look at the big picture.

I laughed as Suzanne told me her exercise and scale story. Tuesday she was 144 pounds, did her step routine then weighed herself again to find out she was 142 pounds. Officially, she is 144 pounds, not 142, I told her.

"Do I wanna go lower? Do I have what it takes?" Suzanne is exercising and drinking water so she knows the extra weight is coming from her food portions.

She was so busy talking that she hardly touched her mocha. This woman sitting across the table from me has changed since January.

We talked about the new step routine. "It's good, hard! I used the easy step routine as the warm-up, did the new one two times then the other routine one time." The "easy" routine was the first one I had given her and it was difficult back then. She feels her heart rate is coming down quicker, which is a good sign.

"It's still hard to go downstairs in the evenings to exercise with the ball but I'm doing it. I can imagine that in the future I might use going into the basement as an excuse not to exercise." To help her, the next routine will be one she can do upstairs.

"When I get tired of doing push-ups on the ball, I like the fact that I can go to the floor. And I might try doing a straight-leg push-up on the floor to see how far down I can get." This is serious progress from the woman who said she couldn't do a push-up.

"I'm a pleaser. I know that." What an interesting statement. I don't see Suzanne trying to please me but I do see her as someone who wants to cross the task off her To Do List.

When Kris opened up a bag of BBQ kettle chips last night, Suzanne said, "It isn't fair. I freaking hate you!" She talked about the smell of the BBQ and how she could have had one, but she didn't have any. Instead, she went downstairs and worked out. "I could have been 144 pounds today if I had eaten the chips."

"I love to swim!" Good, Suzanne will be adding this to the already long list of exercise activities she likes to do. I shocked her by saying that swimming does not count toward her cardio workout. "The heck with that!" I explained that a casual swim will work her heart and lungs but it's not a cardio workout in the same way that intense stepping is. "If I had the choice of sitting in a chair on my butt reading a book versus being in the pool with my children, I'd opt for the pool."

We discussed biking and I explained that a leisurely ride with Ian is not a cardio workout. It is a cardio workout when she's peddling up hills, riding in a higher gear and pushing herself.

Again she talked about her weight. "The 130s—just to smell it—just to go down that low." Her May goals will tell me what Suzanne really wants to do. Right now she is struggling with her weight. There is a direct correlation with it and the fact that she will have to eat less food. Fortunately, confidence is on her side.

Suzanne talked about lessons learned from label-reading. Since our fiber cereal talk, she focused on the cranberry fiber cereal containing nine grams of fiber, so she bought it. When she got it home, she was disappointed to discover that it contains 18 grams of sugar, six more grams than her children's cereal and 15 more than puffed rice. Yes, the cranberry fiber cereal contains a lot of sugar, but if this is the only really sugary item she's having all day, then she's okay. Suzanne definitely understands the importance of sugar and a healthy breakfast when she said, "We have weekend cereal and school cereal."

After the birth of one of her sons, she took him into the office and everyone commented on how good she looked. "That feeling of feeling thin, I want it again! I want to see what the 130s feel like. Getting into the 140s was HUGE!"

A while ago I had talked about having a maximum weight and not going beyond it. Suzanne actually said she might want that number to be 140.

After getting a big bear hug, we parted. Was her shirt tucked in?

Saturday, April 28

Suzanne's Journal Notes ...

"6:00 p.m., ball routine—we're going out tonight and I definitely didn't want to have to worry about the exercise when I got home."

Talk about planning; Suzanne did her ball routine before going out Saturday evening.

Monday, April 30

Suzanne's Journal Notes ...

"I don't know how to explain what I have been feeling today. I went ahead and weighed myself this morning and I didn't like what I saw—144 again. When I look at what I ate over the weekend I understand it, but right now I am not sure I can go to the next level. I know I feel MUCH better in my clothes and the only time I am really not happy is when I look at myself without clothes on. I want to be able to eat a small piece of cake on a Sunday night and not worry about what the scale is going to say the next day. I know there is so much more to learn, so I don't want to give up, but I have obviously hit a roadblock between my love of food and losing weight. We also had Kyle and his kids over yesterday from about 1:30 to 8:30 p.m., so I did not get a walk or bike ride in on such a beautiful day."

The scale might have set Suzanne's mood, but she did say she feels better in her clothes. She struggles with the scale versus her love of food. Her dedication will pay off but it will take time. Hang in there, Suzanne. Be patient but be persistent.

April was another month of firsts for Suzanne: working out while on vacation, wearing a bikini and showing more skin. Ian even complimented Suzanne on her bikini. There was no mention of GERD so we might have corrected that with morning workouts. She's more confident, she's tucking in her shirt, is keeping a journal, exercising and drinking water. She even made it through tax season. But Suzanne is struggling with self-doubt over losing more weight and her love of food.

TO DO:

1. Continue to keep your journal

2. Focus on the positive

3. Plan, plan, plan

May:
The Life-Changing Event

Wednesday, May 2

When I arrived at Suzanne's house, I was greeted by cute little Ian and lovable Tucker the dog. Suzanne was there too, and gave me a long hug.

She talked about the big party they're hosting for her cousin's wedding rehearsal. In preparation for the party she's starting to fix up the house and think about the food she will serve. Suzanne wants to cook for the party but Kris wants it catered so Suzanne can relax.

Suzanne, Ian, Tucker and I went into the basement. Tucker assumed his position on the couch while Ian played with his toys. Suzanne said she might get a small full-length mirror down there so she is able to see her form while she exercises.

She's now 143 pounds and by the way she told me her weight, I asked if she is okay with that. She talked about it being a battle, but when she puts on her clothes she can say, "Yeah. This is great; I love the way my clothes fit!"

"I'd really like to be in the 130s, but I really want the chocolate cake upstairs." To lose weight, Suzanne realizes she has to cut back on portions and exercise a bit more.

"I don't know what my May goals are." Suzanne seemed truly frustrated by that.

Suzanne met her April cardio goal by exercising at least six days a week. She also met her daily water and fruit consumption goal. Regarding her original goal of being comfortable in her own skin, she told me that she is.

"I'm certainly not done, though." Suzanne feels there's more to do and learn but she's struggling. She is proud of what she's accomplished in four months and doesn't focus on what she can't have. "Can I still be in the 130s and have chocolate cake?" That statement explains her struggle.

Suzanne asked what I do when other clients stall. We go back to the basics and I ask the client what she wants to accomplish. Then we figure out a way to get there, just like we're doing with Suzanne.

We continued talking about the struggle of exercising more and eating cake. It's a trade-off because the ultimate goal is to lose weight. Suzanne doesn't know what she wants so she needs to take the next week to figure it out. She does need to make some decisions or she'll be sitting on the fence for a while.

"Since tax season is over, I've mentally relaxed." Suzanne ate lunch at home and had some chocolate cake. If she had gone to work, she would not have packed the cake. This let me know that idle time is dangerous for Suzanne. As a CPA, she was busy during tax season. Now she needs to keep busy and fortunately, planning the rehearsal dinner will help her do that.

I asked again what she wants but she didn't know how to answer yet.

"I've exceeded my expectations but I feel it's too soon to be done! I'll take those pictures on Friday and say 'yikes!' and won't be happy. Would you?"

I reminded her that she talked about getting her weight down to the 130s, so she owes it to herself to get there. She could set a goal to weigh 139 by the end of June, which would mean losing four pounds in two months—about a half-pound a week. "That's doable!" I don't want her to continue to be unsure and to always wonder about the 130s. Suzanne said again she's happy where she is at 143, which is awesome! Still, she didn't seem completely convinced. She tried on a pair of pants from a year ago and they were too big. "I felt thin wearing them."

More than once Kris has said to her, "You're glowing"—and she feels she is—she does feel better.

Kris has been very supportive of Suzanne's journey. This has surprised her because she thought she would get some opposition. He likes buying her clothes and now they fit, when before they didn't.

This conversation took place in less than 30 minutes and would have gone on longer but Suzanne had to take Ian to the bus stop. When she returned she told me that she had found some high-fiber cereal clusters. She ate some this morning and hoped the fiber wouldn't take effect during our boxing session. If it does, she will learn a valuable lesson, like she learned about not eating a heavy meal so close to exercising.

We went back to her goals and she said, "I'm struggling with that. I don't want to be on the fence. In order to achieve weight loss I'm going to have to give something up." Here it was again, that internal struggle from the woman who loves food.

Doing cardio and drinking water are habits now; they don't have to be goals. I suggested she be creative and think of other things that could be a goal. And since she's currently walking, playing tennis and biking, she could cut back to three times a week on her step routine.

Suzanne talked about an elliptical machine and how she'd love to get one. "I could possibly get Kris on it. I deserve it. I want it." She also talked about the bike stand and that she wanted to get one but hasn't because she's been exercising outside. We've already been together through winter and Suzanne reiterated, "I'm not worried about the winter."

We talked about clothes and I suggested that instead of using a number on the scale, maybe she could use fitting into an article of clothing as a goal. Suzanne may have something in her closet that doesn't fit, which she can look forward to wearing.

Referring to four days of not journaling, Suzanne said, "I lost it a little bit but got back on track." I asked if a goal could be not to write down what she eats. "I'm not ready to do that." She wants to journal in the future about feelings instead of writing about what she eats and drinks.

I asked if doing something with Kris could be a May goal. She mentioned that she wants to walk with him. They could take a stroll—not a power walk like she does with her friends, but a time to hold hands and talk. I also suggested that she could have a personal goal that she doesn't have to share with me.

We talked for over an hour; it was important for Suzanne to clear her mind. There was indecision and confusion and she needed some direction. I'll be eager to see what her May goals are.

For kick boxing, we used an '80s CD and she recognized the songs. I picked up the pace and her breathing was entirely different from the last time; I could hardly hear it. Her heart and lungs are getting conditioned.

Suzanne was still struggling with her goals for May. To help her put things in perspective, I told her she had homework for our next meeting. She's to think back to January and list any changes she's made in her life including eating, drinking, exercise, thinking, family, friends, siblings, clothes size, etc. This list should include things that are different from when we started working together in January and can be both positive and negative. It's to be all about her. This will force Suzanne to think about how her life has changed, mostly for the better. It will be an excellent tool to reference when we stop working together.

Friday, May 4

I received an email with "Update" as the subject:

> "Hi Linda, Just a quick update—go figure, I was 141 this morning. And after exercise, just for fun, I was JUST under the 140 marker. It feels good today. I'll have my homework and goals for Wednesday. See you then. Suz P.S. Enjoy this beautiful weather. I'll be in Lancaster at a soccer tournament all day tomorrow."

I sent her a congratulatory email saying she knows what being in the 130s feels like then shared my good news; I just learned that I won the Women's Referral Network–MacElree Harvey award. (This is an initiative award created by the law firm MacElree Harvey and given to a WRN member who has helped promote the WRN and has shown initiative. The winner receives a $750 grant to present to the charity of her choice. In my case, it will go to the Domestic Violence Center, of which I have been a supporter for 20 years.)

She responded via email:

> *"Linda, I wish I could say that I had done the nominating myself, because nobody deserves it more than you! Now I'm already getting emotional about the luncheon and I can't wait to stand up and cheer for all you have done for the WRN (and ME!!!). See you then. Suz"*

When I think about this Tuesday's WRN luncheon, instead of thinking about the award, I get excited knowing Suzanne is going to be there looking amazing and feeling confident. Another exciting thing is that my parents will be there. Yes, it is a women's organization but a few men attend. Mom was a regular when I was the president of the organization but Dad's never been to a meeting. The other exciting thing is that Tuesday, May 8—the day of the luncheon—is Mom and Dad's 53rd wedding anniversary. They were going to go out to lunch to celebrate but changed their plans (when they heard I won) so Mom could attend the luncheon. With parents like that, I had to invite Dad. The award is nice but knowing that Suzanne—who will look radiant, and my parents—on their 53rd wedding anniversary—will be there, means more to me.

Suzanne's Journal Notes …

> *"8:00 p.m. Saturday, May 5: Tom's 40th birthday party. I had one margarita, a beer and at least 20 ounces of water. I ate three tortilla chips with salsa, one wienie wrap, one mini-quiche and about 10 Swedish fish."*

Parties equate to lots of alcohol and food. Instead of eating and drinking the night away, Suzanne kept track.

Tuesday, May 8

I was at the WRN 20th Anniversary Luncheon early, helping them set up, when I saw Suzanne. She has an infectious smile. My parents were with me so I introduced her to Dad; she already knew Mom from previous luncheons. We hugged hi and I asked her how much weight she'd lost. "Sixteen pounds but it was 15 this morning." So we all agreed that it was 16 pounds. She looked cute, which she always does. She told us her May goal was to run a half-mile; she thought a mile was too aggressive. Since Suzanne and I were meeting the next day, I suggested we run. There was a look of shock on her face but she agreed to do it. Mom and Dad were witnesses to the fact that Suzanne would be running tomorrow.

Wednesday, May 9

When I pulled in Suzanne's driveway, she was getting her bike out. Ian and Tucker were also in the driveway—they were the welcoming committee.

We sat at the kitchen table and talked about running when Ian said, "Mom, you can't run!" She quickly said, "Linda thinks I can!"

She handed me her May photos and said she was smiling, not because she likes having her picture taken, but because of what Kris had said. Which was? "Holy cow!"

Referring to the difference between last month's and this month's photos, Suzanne said, "I still don't see it." I showed her the January photos and she blurted, "Oh, I look fat!" When Suzanne looked at the photos she commented, "I still can't get rid of the back rolls." I explained that it was fatty tissue and that running would help redefine her body. "This is just humiliating," she said about having her picture taken in bike pants and a sports bra. I said we'd take pictures of her at the end of June in her January clothing. Then she'll see a dramatic difference, because with stretchy clothes like the bike pants, she can't see too much of a change. When she drops a size or two, she will see the difference.

I asked how she was feeling. "Good, definitely good! Yesterday I weighed 142 and I didn't weigh myself today. Tuesday's number was my weight from the weekend and Friday's is what I've done during the week."

How did she feel after boxing? "A few places in my back were tight but they didn't linger."

I asked about her May goals, which she had written down:

– Jog at least ½ mile

– Weight at 140

– Continue to get fruit in every day because it's not a habit. I'm not a huge berry person. (She's to eat fruits she likes. She loves pineapple but said it contains sugar. I told her that it's okay to eat pineapple—everything in moderation.)

– Catching up on paperwork. I want my wallet cleaned out by the end of the month. (She has debit receipts in there and can't get her wallet closed.) This one isn't exercise-or food-related. Since Christmas I'm so far behind.

– Wedding thing. The rehearsal dinner is at our house. Experience through the process. The joy of the occasion is something I want to feel without having to worry about the food. I used to care about what the hors d'oeuvres would be and now I want to worry about Aunt Susie.

Her homework was to list both positives and negatives she's experienced since starting her journey in January. She had her list and even told my parents yesterday that she had her homework done.

Here is her list:

POSITIVES:

– Exercise has been in my life every day since January 5 and has become part of my routine

– I've lost 16 pounds

– Everything I own that I have tried on either fits or is too big

- The wonderful support from Kris

- The positive comments from friends

- Definitely happier

- I know it's possible for me to lose weight without giving up the foods that I love

- I know it's possible for me to find the time to exercise

"There are a hundred more," she said of the positives but she wrote down eight.

NEGATIVES:

- Getting up at 5:45 a.m.

- I'll have to have my pants altered

I told Suzanne to look at the list next year, when we're not working together. If she's gotten off track, this list will help her get back on track.

"My mom's a complete inspiration. I never thought about it till the first lunch we had. That has been so meaningful. If she can do it, I can do it. I've got part of her genes." I told Suzanne I never know what I'll say will stick with a client and this one about her mom certainly did.

I brought over empty snack food packages, wanting to show Suzanne some examples of choices she could make. Ian was sitting at the table with us and thought food was in the boxes—he was most interested in the ice cream. When she read the ingredients on the Lean Pockets package, she said she could read them because the ingredients weren't mostly unpronounceable chemicals. She's not into preservatives, which is good.

Suzanne had already informed me that, "I can't eat just a frozen entree because I like to eat more than one thing."

Her family used to have pizza once a week and now she doesn't really crave it. If they do have it, she'll have one slice instead of two but she often opts to cook a quick meal rather than order pizza. That's a serious change in taste.

When she chooses daily foods, if she's already consumed a lot of sodium, she shouldn't eat salty pretzels. We also discussed white flour, which many foods contain.

I showed her a box of Cracker Jacks, which we used to have when we were younger. "This has less sugar than that darn cereal I just bought." Lesson learned. Look at the nutritional labels.

Suzanne asked if almonds would be a good snack. Absolutely, and I suggested she pack them since stores typically don't sell single- serving sizes.

When we finished discussing food choices and labels I asked if she was ready to run. "Yes, as ready as I'll ever be."

It was 65 degrees outside, sunny, no breeze—a perfect day to run. We made a left turn out of her driveway and walked to the stop sign, then I told her to start running while I rode her bike. She had a slow, steady jog just above a fast walk and seemed comfortable with it. I kept talking to her and checking her feet, making sure she wasn't running on her toes or rolling to one side of her foot. "The park entrance is around four mailboxes up." Suzanne thought we were running to the park but I told her to run to the stop sign at the end of the street. As we neared the park, Suzanne started to cry. I asked if she was okay and wondered if she had pulled a muscle. No, they were tears of joy, so I high-fived her. She didn't tell me this till later: at the park entrance she realized she had just run a half-mile, which had been her goal.

Suzanne ran past the park and to the end of the street. When we got to the stop sign I touched the sign with my hand and told her to do the same. She smacked it and thought we were stopping. No, I told her to run back home and to slow down her pace or walk if she got tired.

On the way back home, Suzanne's breathing was excellent, which meant she had a good pace. "I guess I need another goal!"

As we neared her driveway I let her know she had been running for 19 minutes. Did she want to go for 20 or stop? She wanted to stop but when she got in the driveway she kept jogging in place. "Tell me when it's 20." I got off the bike and had her jog with me down the street till my watch hit 20 minutes.

When I told her it was 20 minutes, Suzanne threw both hands up in the air, let out a loud—I don't know what it was— a scream, a yell, a woo-hoo—and then she started to sob. I got the biggest hug and we stood there in the street hugging and jumping up and down. She had just run 20 minutes. "I never would have done this without you," she said through her tears.

We walked down the street and I kept rubbing Suzanne's back, telling her she had done it. She was still crying. "Thirty years ago I got cut by the lacrosse team. You don't know what this means to me. Why didn't I think I couldn't do it? I know that's a double negative." I explained that I see the potential in people and part of my job is to help them see it, then achieve it.

Suzanne had a smile that I've never seen before. Something happened inside her. Something changed. In 20 short minutes she had erased 30 long years of self-doubt. It was a life-changing event for her, powerful and very emotional. We walked to the end of her street, then back to her house. I was skipping and pumping my fists, telling her she did it. It was amazing to witness!

"Nothing can go wrong today!" I really believed Suzanne when she said that.

While running, we talked about the slope of the road and I reiterated it on our walk back to the house—she should be sure to run with a different leg on the down slope of the road. I showed her, as we were walking, how our right leg is longer and our left leg is shorter. If we came back on the opposite side of the road, our right leg would be longer and our left leg shorter. She should watch the slope of the road so she doesn't throw her body out of alignment.

We stretched on her deck while talking about the importance of staying hydrated. I also explained the importance of walking to warm up, doing a light jog, walking to cool down and then stretching.

We concentrated the stretches on her calves and quads. I told her to keep stretching her leg muscles throughout the day and suggested she wear flat shoes instead of heels because she hadn't jogged in 30 years. She's to keep drinking water, too. I asked her to wait 48 hours to see how she felt, then jog again if she wanted to. She talked about the bar being set at 20 minutes but I explained that she might not always have 20 minutes to run or feel like running 20 minutes. She should listen to her body.

"I can't wait to call Kris!"

As I was leaving Suzanne said, "I know you are going to clock the route then email me how long it is."

"I have the best trainer!" After Suzanne said this, I was thinking that I have the best client because I knew she could run a half-mile and she just proved it. Her run will stay with me forever—her tears of joy and erasing years of self-doubt. It still gives me chills.

I clocked our route and came up with 1.4 miles, which blew her half-mile goal right out of the water.

At our next meeting, I'll suggest Suzanne try a one-mile fun run race. She can do it and she might just incorporate the family into the event.

People say I must be proud of what I've done for Suzanne but you're continuing to read that it's Suzanne who does the work and takes the initiative to do more. I'm proud of her gain in self-confidence, which has an impact on every part of her life. Oh, what's next?

Suzanne's Journal Notes …

"I couldn't wait to share my story with Kris and thank goodness he was available for lunch. We shared a quesadilla and each had the salad bar and water and he enjoyed my story. I am so proud of myself and Kris was, too. I really am starting to think that Kris would like to do something too. He asked me if Linda has male clients and I told him about Lenny. Lenny lost 100 pounds while

*working with Linda. Kris and I talked about my lack of
confidence when Linda and I started working together
and that somehow Linda directed me down a path of
success. I do not want to push Kris, but I hope he decides
to take a step."*

Saturday, May 12

Suzanne's Journal Notes ...

*"8:00 a.m. on Sat., May 12, I was lying in bed on this
magnificent morning when I decided that if I was ever
going to try and run again, it should be now. So I got
myself out of bed and did the same run again. It was
so beautiful outside. My body wasn't nearly as sore this
morning. On my return trip Kris and KJ passed me on
their way to soccer. I got the best 'go mom' and 'keep
it up hon' that I felt like I could run forever. Their smiles
were filled with such genuine pride that it really motivated
me to want to continue. From the run it was on to Ian's
baseball pictures and game. I didn't have time for a
shower; oh well, the folks at the ball field were just going
to have to take me for what I was. I have to say that
staying in my running clothes kept reminding me over and
over about what an accomplishment I did that morning."*

Sunday, May 13

Suzanne's Journal Notes ...

*"Mother's Day, May 13th! Breakfast: 8:30 a.m. I had my
standard bowl of cereal. Kris and the boys surprised me
with cards, plants from the boys and a beautiful new ring
from Kris. He really doesn't believe in Mother's Day for
me because I am not his mother but for some reason, this
year he really surprised me. The ring is gorgeous—spoiled
again! We had a terrific family tennis outing at the park.
KJ and I paired up against Kris and Griffin. We beat them*

pretty easily (KJ did most of the work) and then Griffin and I played four games of singles and he beat me three games to one. It was so fun to be out there together. Ian played a little and then went over to the playground—the beauty of the park."

Thursday, May 17

I arrived at Suzanne's house before 8:00 a.m. and Ian said I could come in. He was dressed for school with his little knapsack on his back. Suzanne gave me a big hug and Tucker was there to greet me, too.

I met Kris. We all listened to Ian talk about the wedding. He has to wear "pointy shoes," which he wasn't too thrilled about. Ian kept saying he wanted to show me his outfit, a tux.

As we stood in the kitchen Kris and I were standing shoulder to shoulder. He put an arm around me and half hugged me while saying, "Thank you for what you did for my wife. She smiles more." We both continued to give Suzanne compliments and I agreed that she does look good. Kris was truly proud of her and liked the new Suzanne.

After Suzanne ran with me on Wednesday she had sore legs for a few days. When she ran Saturday, she had sore legs for a day. Then, when she ran Monday, she hardly had sore legs. These are signs that her legs are getting used to jogging. What I didn't like was her neck pain. Her neck had been sore, right at the base of it on the right side and some in her mid-back. When she turned her head to the right, she could feel it in her neck. She said the pain in her back might be stress. I asked that she keep an eye on this pain.

I told her it might be a good idea for her to carry pepper spray on morning jogs. Yes, at 6:00 a.m. she should be aware of her surroundings and should carry her cell phone and ID. I suggested she take extra time before jogging to warm up—do the step routine for a few minutes, push-ups or walk a little bit farther before starting to run.

I asked her about entering a race and she laughed. "That's so funny. My neighbor said that. I won't rule it out. The neighbor, who ran a race with her family, said the race would keep me motivated to work out."

We talked about Suzanne possibly running when her family goes to the Outer Banks this summer. She asked about sand and I told her I'm not a fan of running on it because of the slope and how hard it can be on the calves. If she's on compact sand or on a boardwalk, she'll be fine.

We talked about running shoes, which will give her forward and back support, versus cross-trainers, which will give her that plus lateral support. If Suzanne intends to run miles on a regular basis, she should invest in good running sneaks. We talked about walking sneaks too. Because Suzanne wants to do a little bit of everything, she'll purchase cross-trainers.

We had just started working out when her neighbor Kathy stopped by with the most beautifully decorated cookies I've ever seen. Kathy said to me, "I've heard a lot about you."

We finally got back to working out and I commented on Suzanne's balance, how good it was. "Balance, that's improved. That's definitely improved. I noticed it in the shower shaving my legs." It's not just the scale that is showing Suzanne results, it's something as basic as shaving her legs.

I had given Suzanne a handled exercise tube that she'd be able to take on vacation like she did the brown bands. I want her to keep thinking that exercise doesn't stop just because she's on vacation. I also gave Suzanne a routine for the new exercise tube. As she took me through the moves she said proudly, "I didn't even look at my notes." She was catching on quickly and her form was excellent. "That feels good. I might put it in my briefcase and do some exercises during the day!"

Suzanne talked about the reverse curls, the ones she hated and thought she couldn't do. "I love those now!" When we were done she said, "Awesome!"

Later that day I sent Suzanne an email suggesting Kris ride the bike while she ran. It would be a great bonding time for them but more importantly, he might be able to see something in her body alignment or stride that is irritating her neck.

Friday, May 18

Suzanne's Journal Notes …

"Wedding Day, May 18th: I have to admit that I slept in and did not do my step this morning. I knew I would do a lot of dancing later, so I hope that counts.

"Breakfast and lunch were typical then I think I snuck in a leftover cookie bar or two. It's not good having all the great leftovers in the house!

"Appetizers and dinner started at 6:00 p.m. One fried shrimp, one spanakopita, two beef rolls and two stuffed mushrooms. I had three sea breezes and two glasses of champagne throughout the evening. For dinner I ate 2/3 of my filet, two bites of the stuffed potato, roll and all of the green beans and carrots. I never saw my dessert, which is a good thing because I had enough at home! There was SO much food out and available all weekend, but with so many people around there were plenty of stories to enjoy along with the food. And therefore, there was less emphasis on the food."

There were certain special events that happened during Suzanne's journey and this was one of them. In January she would have focused on the food and now, in May, she focused on the occasion. Suzanne still has a love for food but has slowly detached from it.

Wednesday, May 23

Tucker was there to greet me when I got to Suzanne's house. "He's a leaner." Yes he is, because he nearly knocked me over.

We went toward the basement but Suzanne didn't want to go down there. "It smells like dirty kids and stale farts." She cracks me up with some of her statements.

We sat at the dining room table to look at wedding pictures. Suzanne has one attractive family! The sons I haven't met, KJ and Griffin, are tall. Suzanne's outfit was gorgeous. I asked how she felt. "Fantastic!"

KJ's birthday is today and he wanted Hamburger Helper for dinner then strawberries and cream and a cookie concoction for dessert. Suzanne took it as a compliment, indicating she's such a good cook that her children want Hamburger Helper for their birthday.

"I was 141 this morning and it's not a weigh-in morning. I had a major victory Monday night, which was our anniversary. It was 8:30 p.m. when Kris said he wanted to go to the Cheesecake Factory for dinner. The menu caused a challenge for me—it took a while to order. Remember, I read cookbooks for enjoyment! I decided on a chicken wrap appetizer for my dinner. I only got one thing."

Over the weekend Suzanne felt really stressed because she hadn't exercised, so on Sunday she ran while Ian biked with her. I asked if she still had the neck pain. "No, I still feel like I'm tight though. I feel you hit the nail on the head with it being a chilly early morning." Suzanne is learning how to warm up, literally.

She asked if I know when a client was going to make it and be successful. Yes. Everyone has the potential and having fitness as a priority is very important. Suzanne has made it a priority to exercise daily and to keep a daily journal. There is a correlation between that and her success.

"People ask me, 'How'd you do it?' and I say 'Linda does something. She works some type of magic.'" My "magic" was asking Suzanne what her goals were then taking a journey to achieve them.

We talked about alcoholism, addiction, obesity, family issues and all the different things that play a part in who we are. Childhood is important too, because things happen back then and if a situation isn't dealt with, it comes forward into our adult life. I shared a story with Suzanne about a former client who was sexually abused as a young child. The client didn't know how to deal with the situation so she ate it, literally, till she weighed over 300 pounds.

We changed gears and I had her show me her new handled strap exercises. While doing the abductor exercise she said, "This one's the hardest one. I should have beautiful hips when I'm done."

Suzanne likes having the strap to use upstairs instead of having to go into the basement each night to use the ball. Exercise needs to be convenient so she has no excuses.

Suzanne talked about the tennis banquet. "Being the vain person that I am, I thought 'What cute outfit can I wear?' But I ended up wearing what I had on—shorts, top and sneaks—so I was ready to work out if the opportunity were to arise. I NEVER would have done that before."

Suzanne always dresses up when she sees clients but recently she went wearing her workout clothes. The client said, "You look beautiful! You've lost a lot of weight." Suzanne laughed because she was wearing sneaks, shorts and an athletic top.

We practiced new step moves and it was funny to see Suzanne using her fingers to keep track of the repetitions. "I'm an accountant!" I asked about her breathing and recovery time doing Fast Feet. "I definitely notice a quicker recovery in Fast Feet." In the past she'd have to stop to get a drink before and sometimes after Fast Feet, but not now.

I asked about her May goals. "We beat the running goal already. Paperwork: no. Weight: I'm hovering. I can't remember the other one." Fruit? "I'm doing well. I'm happy. Can you tell? I think I was smiling watching TV last night."

I want to bottle her feelings and pass them out to the rest of the folks on a journey to fitness. Imagine feeling this happy. She's in control of her life and I know she won't go back to 157 pounds.

Thursday, May 24

Suzanne's Journal Notes ...

"6:00 a.m., 25 minutes of step. I did a warm-up and then ran through Linda's new routine three times. I really like the new step routine, but I think my legs may be tired from all the squats. After dinner I took KJ to soccer practice. It was a beautiful night and I felt like being outside, so I wore my jogging clothes and went for a 20-minute run while KJ had practice. I ran around the outside of the soccer field, on the grass. Beth and Pat were there for Connor's lacrosse game, so when I was finished I stopped to say hello to everyone. It felt really good to run! The weather was absolutely perfect. I got over feeling like a dork in front of the two soccer dads and the boys practicing."

What a momentous occasion for Suzanne—to jog someplace other than the comfort of her neighborhood and to jog in front of strangers and friends.

Saturday, May 26

Suzanne's Journal Notes...

"We had barbecued chicken thighs, shrimp antipasto and fresh fruit. I didn't eat any bread, but Nat made a wonderful banana-coconut cream dessert and I had quite a piece. Kyle came for dinner. After dinner we set up for games. We all played Taboo (kids too!). For games they put out cookies, veggies, trail mix and pretzels. I couldn't eat a thing. I was full from dinner. I only drank water and laughed a ton during the game."

It appears to be mandatory to serve snacks when we play games. Because whatever is offered gets eaten, I'd like to see a tray of fruits and veggies served. In this case, Suzanne made a conscious choice not to eat the snacks. When people are in that type of social situation they have a tendency to lose track of the food they eat and the alcohol they drink. Suzanne is keeping a journal so she knows she has to record anything she consumes. She eliminated mindless eating.

Wednesday, May 30

Suzanne's Journal Notes ...

"6:00 a.m., 26 minutes of step. After two days of 'detox' (as I call it), my weight finally came down. I guess I really needed to get all of the yummy summer foods out of the way so I could get back on track. I have noticed that I am starting to see a pattern with my eating. I seem to eat pretty big over the weekends and then more responsibly during the week. If I can do that and keep my weight under control, I will be a happy camper."

Like clockwork, Suzanne's body responded to her cutting back on what she ate.

Thursday, May 31

I arrived at Suzanne's house with a wiffle bat and a bag of hard plastic balls in my hand.

"Officially 140. I sort of stepped on the scale like this," Suzanne proclaimed as she proceeded to tiptoe onto a pretend scale.

I went right into her May goals. Goal Number One: Jog at least a half-mile? "Check." We were interrupted when Ian came into the room and saw the wiffle bat and balls. I asked if he'd help me by pitching the balls to his mom every day so she can hit them right-handed and then left-handed. Ian asked, "Who will pick up the balls, you? Are we doing it now?" I explained that his mom could pick up the balls because it will be exercise for her and we can't do it now because he has a school bus to catch. When I told him the bat and balls were theirs, he said, "We get to keep them?"

We went back to Suzanne's goals:

Number Two: Weight 140? "Check."

Number Three: Fruit daily? "Yes. It's not one-hundred percent each day unless you count raisins in my cereal." Raisins in cereal don't count.

Number Four: Catch up on paperwork? "I'm working on it."

I asked how she's doing with the new step moves. "Great, love them! I used to get winded after Fast Feet and even more winded after squats. Now, I'm not as winded." She did all four step routines twice and it took about 25 minutes. "The first one is a warm-up." Great progress because the first routine is where she started.

"I have fun things to tell you from the weekend." She stayed with friends and tried to eat healthy snacks in the afternoon, ate dinner, and then had no snacks while playing games "because I was full from dinner, so it was easy to say no." This is a powerful statement—the ability to say no. She is in control.

Her second fun thing was about birthday cake. "My favorite breakfast is leftover store-bought birthday cake—the sheet cake." Her friend was going to give her some cake to bring home but Suzanne said no. Suzanne turned down birthday cake because she knew that if she brought it home, she'd eat it for breakfast. If the cake is not here, she can't eat it. Perfect—eliminate temptation.

When we met in January Suzanne told me she hates to throw out food; the third fun thing dealt with this. Some of the food and sodas from the rehearsal dinner had to be thrown out and she felt badly about it. But as she said, "I can't eat it," so she threw it out. Suzanne is learning to do what is best for her.

We talked about our working together. I'm glad we are because Suzanne gets to see how I operate and more importantly, Suzanne gets to feel things—intangible things. Over the last five months she has experienced the tangible effects of losing weight, drinking more water and exercising: her clothes fit better and she has more energy. But what's more important are her feelings. She feels more in control, more confident, more successful and better about herself. No one can give Suzanne these feelings; she has to get them herself.

"I'm happy. I'm so much happier!"

"My morning energy is great and the night is okay." Nights are more sedentary and the family will put on the TV, which is not what Suzanne wants. "I like to walk or do something after dinner to get away from it."

Suzanne shared a good story with me. One evening the kids were in the family room; the TV was on but it seemed like they wanted to talk. She asked that the TV be turned off and sure enough, they had a wonderful family conversation.

Tucker was barking at the back door so Suzanne let him in. "He gets jealous and he's a mama's boy." Tucker came over to where Suzanne was sitting, put a paw on each shoulder and proceeded to lick and hug her. After a few licks and hugs, he was fine and quietly walked away. If you count Tucker, Suzanne has four boys.

I asked about Tucker running with her. "When I walk him I get shin splints." If walking the dog gives Suzanne shin splints, running with him is definitely out of the question. She's too new to running—we don't want her messing up any body parts.

"The month really snuck up on me." Suzanne realizes that without goals, the month would be gone. Because she had a daily and a monthly goal, she stayed on track and didn't lose the month of May.

After we finished talking, we went outside into the gorgeous 75-degree weather. For something different, we turned right and walked to the stop sign. Suzanne thought we were going to keep walking but I had her turn around and start to jog. It was a slow pace, one foot in front of the other. I asked her to make a right and the surprise on her face let me know she knew there was a hill, a decent-size hill. I could hear a little breath but not too much, so that was a good sign. She commented that it was a big hill and it was, considering she'd never run up one that size before. At the next street, I had her make a right. This hill was bigger and longer. Suzanne was catching onto my pattern and said, "The next hill is even longer!" She was correct. Suzanne commented about her heel so I watched her form and it was fine.

Suzanne figured I already had measured the distance of this new route and I would have if she were running a race but since she's not, this route is about time and technique.

When we were on flat ground, two different times I had Suzanne run faster. At this new pace, she has a beautiful runner's stride. During our outing, I didn't want to push her too hard but just enough so she could feel what it's like to run up hills and run at a faster pace, referred to as intervals. The run took 22 minutes and her breathing was fine, which tells me she was running at a comfortable pace. She did an amazing job and has now added two more choices to her jog: hills and intervals.

Suzanne said her June goals should include running, maybe twice a week. I asked her to wait 48 hours before running again and she asked in a panic, "Can I step?" Yes, but wait 48 hours before running again, then choose either hills or intervals, not both. Slow and steady.

"I like order and routine in my life and now my routine is thrown off." Suzanne was talking about work slowing down, the kids would be out of school soon and summer activities would start. Her current routine would be thrown off so she needed to create a new routine for summer. Two words have helped her to be successful in her journey: order and routine.

Tugging on her shorts she said, "My first official size 8 and all the size 8s I tried on fit. I was a 10 for a really, really long time." Suzanne now has to get her pants altered. This and buying smaller clothes makes her accountable to her wardrobe. If she gains weight, the clothes go back to the tailor to be let out...I don't think so.

During May Suzanne battled the feeling that she had stalled in her progress. She struggled with eating chocolate cake versus losing more weight. To help her, she made a list of both positive and negative things that had happened to her since she started her journey. A life-changing experience happened on May 9 when Suzanne jogged. This emotional 20-minute jog erased 30 years of self-doubt. She continued to experience triumphs but none as monumental as her jog.

To Do:

1. Pick a goal that you think might be way out there, then figure out how to achieve it

2. List the positives and negatives from the time you started your journey

---

June:

Adjusting the Routine

Saturday, June 2

Suzanne's Journal Notes ...

"7:00 a.m., I went for a very brisk walk with Carol, Caitlin and Teresa—my fitness friends! They walked so fast. I should have warmed up more. We walked to the park and did both loops, and then we did the first loop two more times—about five miles in about an hour and 15 minutes. On the way home Carol and I jogged from the park exit to her house. Unfortunately, I didn't wear my good sports bra, and I think due to the way I was supporting myself, I stretched my back funny."

Monday, June 4

Suzanne's Journal Notes ...

"6:00 a.m., 27 minutes of step. I didn't sleep very well last night. I started to get stressed about money again. It seems to be feast or famine with us. We have been living high on the hog since Kris got his bonus and then also exercised some stock options. But the reality is that summer is right around the corner and I am not going to be getting a regular paycheck. Even though my paycheck isn't big, it still really helps out. And we still have things we really want to buy. I promised Kris we would get the deck furniture. I didn't realize how expensive the furniture was going to be, but now we have to figure it out."

Money affects Suzanne's sleep but doesn't cause her to eat.

Tuesday, June 5

Suzanne's Journal Notes ...

"6:00 a.m., 25 minutes of step. After my workout I decided to weigh myself again to see if by any chance I had dipped down into the 130s before I ate or drank anything. I know the reality, but seeing the lower weight still feels good. But when I got on the scale it said 145! I couldn't figure it out. I moved the scale around, I got up and down on the scale and over and over; it still said 145. What the hell?"

I've suggested that Suzanne step for a different amount of time so her body doesn't get used to 25 minutes each morning at 6:00 a.m. She needs to shock her body and she certainly is doing that. Another shock is the scale going up five pounds. It doesn't make sense and it could have an impact on her day.

Wednesday, June 6

Suzanne's Journal Notes ...

"Well, I figured out what happened with the scale. Kris decided to weigh himself yesterday. I didn't even realize there was a wheel on the scale to make sure the needle is at the zero. I have looked for the wheel, but I never found it. Kris adjusted the wheel when he got on the scale yesterday. I was so mad, because even though our scale may be wrong, at least it was consistent. Now, I don't know how to get it to where it was other than to re-adjust the wheel to wherever gets me back to 140 pounds. I know we have a cheap scale and should buy a better one, but I wanted the scale to at least be consistent through my first six months with Linda.

"Kris and I had our first fitness-related fight. He messed with my scale."

Suzanne used the word "sabotage" because she wasn't sure if Kris had intentionally adjusted the scale. He's been very supportive so this does not seem to be the case, but Suzanne might encounter people who will try to sabotage her; they liked the old Suzanne and might not like this new one.

Friday, June 8

Today we are meeting at a park and I asked Suzanne to meet me at the tennis courts so she'd think we were going to play tennis. When I saw her drive in, I waved her up near the baseball field. "What do I need? Am I scared?"

We looked at her new photos; Suzanne said there's a big difference from January. As I went through the photos, she pointed to her "wrinkly" stomach and where she saw a difference around her shoulders/bra line and waist. Her face looks thinner, too.

Suzanne set the scale to register her weight at 140 and she's 139 this morning. She was hoping to jump up and down with excitement when she finally reached 139, "but I feel it's been discounted."

"I did intervals on Wednesday. I feel the neck episode from May was from not warming up enough."

I asked about her June goals:

- 138

- Finish paperwork

- Jog two times a week

- Continue what I'm doing—eat fruit and exercise daily

- By the end of the month, work out a summer routine. (I really like this one. We're done working with each other at the end of this month, so Suzanne needs to have things in place for the rest of the year. I'd also like to see her try her January daily routine because she'll be shocked to see how easy it is.)

"I've only done the wiffle ball three times and I'm not a bad left-handed hitter. Last night Ian, Griffin and I were out back playing with it and we had fun. I impressed KJ the other night by not only hitting the ball, but also hitting it left-handed. He tried it left-handed and wasn't having much success. KJ said, 'Mom, you're cranking them!'"

We walked to the baseball field; I had a glove that fit her. "I haven't had a glove on in so long. I throw like a girl. Are you going to teach me how to throw?" We threw for a few minutes and she did throw like a girl—too much wrist—so we worked on that. "Oh, I wish KJ were here." We're giving Suzanne the confidence and skills to play sports so she can play them with her boys. "You have to remember I grew up with all women—well, except for my dad."

After throwing and catching, I walked half-way to the mound with eleven hard balls.

Suzanne hit four balls right-handed and seven balls left-handed. She came seriously close to hitting me with a line drive and said, "Oh no, after all you've done for me and I almost hit you!" Her goal was to hit the ball to the grass and my goal was to not get hit by her ball.

I asked Suzanne to hit the ball right-handed then run the bases. The first time she ran to home plate she put both hands up in the air and jumped on the plate. "I never ran past first base before." The second time around the bases she said, "I'm getting winded." We did this five times and she asked if it counted as intervals.

"I'm such an athletic wannabe. I was almost always picked last even though I look athletic."

After a water break, I had Suzanne hitting balls left-handed and running the bases clockwise. This was working her body in the opposite direction. Two people were watching us and we could only imagine what they were thinking—look at those girls running around the bases backwards!

After baseball, we moved to the grassy part of the field. I pulled out orange cones and a soccer ball. Two badminton birdies fell out and Suzanne said, "Is that next week?"

"I've never played soccer before." I put the cones in a line and had her dribble the ball using only her right foot "Oh, my son would be so embarrassed." To balance both sides of her body, Suzanne went down and back using her left foot.

Our final workout was having her try to score a goal on me. We laughed a lot and were dripping in sweat. It was so humid that it felt like 95 degrees, not 75 degrees.

"That was fun. I loved it!" Suzanne is living proof that exercise can be fun.

We talked about running in the winter and I told her she should dress in clothing that she normally would wear for weather about 30 degrees warmer than it was outside. "Your body heats up," and that is exactly what it does.

From her journal she re-capped our sports outing with:

> "The best part is that it is all stuff I can do with the family that doesn't cost us any money."

Tuesday, June 12

Suzanne's Journal Notes ...

"Ian's class did a poetry reading this morning. They all read poems that they wrote. It was so great. I love watching the kids. Then at 12:45 we had a class picnic for them. For the class picnic I knew we were going to be outside, so I packed up some games. I had fun playing with the kids. Instead of just organizing the games like the other moms did, I actually got in the game and played with them. Then the other moms followed suit and played too. We did a three- legged race, an egg race and played

*wiffle ball (thanks Linda, I took some balls and the bat)
and the kids had so much fun, and so did I! I don't think I
would have participated like I did this time last year. I was
disappointed when our time outside with the kids seemed
like it was over too quickly!"*

What an amazing thing—Suzanne participated!

Wednesday, June 13

Suzanne's Journal Notes ...

*"6:00 a.m., 25-minute run. I did some intervals and I ran
farther. I went through another neighborhood and up by
the creek. Once again, it really felt good."*

Suzanne found something she likes to do.

Saturday, June 16

Suzanne's Journal Notes ...

*"Breakfast: 9:00 a.m., corn muffin and a non-fat, no-whip
mocha from the coffee shop. We sat out on the deck and
enjoyed the breakfast. It has to be one of my top ten things
to do—sit out on the deck. It was so beautiful outside, and
the entire world just seems to move a little bit slower at
that time. It really feels like a mini-vacation for me!"*

When I met Suzanne at her house later that morning we decided to
sit on her deck. She showed me a yoga mat, still in its original wrap. "I
never used it and bought it the first week we started."

She explained the kids' sports schedule: Griffin and Ian have swim practice from 5:30-7:00 p.m. and KJ has soccer practice three times a week.
Suzanne is trying to figure out the dinner schedule—when everyone
should eat and what they should eat. "Unlike in my previous life, one
evening I cut a cantaloupe for another side dish."

During one of Suzanne's drive-the-kids-all-over-the-place nights, she ate chicken in the car with her fingers. "You know that meals have to be an event for me." It's true because eating in the car was not an "event" for Suzanne. Because the "event" was not satisfying, she ate another dinner when she got home.

Suzanne said the word that is a reason for her success: routine. "You know I like my routine. The family goes on a strict budget because I cut back at work. I've got lunches to deal with, kids at home, kids to go various places and my list goes on." She needs to go through all of these different events in her life, even sports schedules, so she can help plan for the next time they come up.

Suzanne said recognition is another reason for her success. She recognizes little things, like how she can do something differently. Suzanne also recognizes that she does things now that she didn't do prior to working with me, like having cantaloupe as a side dish for dinner.

"For me, an empty schedule is more dangerous than a full one." This is a part of Suzanne's personality and one that needs to be dealt with. She needs to keep busy.

Tomorrow is Father's Day, so her family is going to Kris's parents' house. "His Italian mom will make homemade sauce and delicious meatballs." Suzanne's plan is to eat more meat, because she likes it, more fruit and less pasta.

I asked her weight and with a half-smile she answered, "139 after I ran."

How did she feel after we played baseball and soccer? "Emotionally, I was on such a high and I told everyone."

We talked about Ian's school picnic. Suzanne smiled as she shared the story and it was obvious the kids had fun playing games with her. "Ian said the kids cheered when my name was picked to go on the next field trip."

"I ran for 30 minutes yesterday. 30, 30, 30, 30," she said while pumping her hands in the air and swirling them around. "I hate to say it, but

I crave it!" For thirty years Suzanne thought she couldn't run and now she ran for thirty minutes.

"People who inspired me along the way include my mom, because she has weighed the same all these years and Caitlin and Carol, my fitness friends. Caitlin's mom is 70 and hikes." Suzanne doesn't realize this, but on her journey, she is inspiring people.

"Somehow everything is a little sweeter. The trees are greener, the sky is bluer…I don't know." Suzanne has gained confidence and self-esteem. She has less turmoil in her life when it comes to how she feels about herself. She won't go back to 157 pounds. She'll keep trying new things and life will get better for her. Success is a motivator!

"Our workout last week was great, great, great!" I didn't realize playing baseball and soccer would have such an impact on her.

Kris and Ian were home from Ian's baseball game. Ian looked adorable in his red and white uniform. As Suzanne was doing a challenging pushup, she said to Kris, "Do I look sexy?" Kris laughed and Ian smirked. They were all going to the baseball picnic, so Suzanne picked up her exercise equipment, hugged me bye, then ran inside.

Sunday, June 17

Suzanne's Journal Notes …

"Father's Day! 9:00 a.m., Kris and I went for the double-loop walk in the park. It was a beautiful morning. It was his idea, and it was marvelous! We walked faster than I thought we would—definitely not a stroll. We didn't even talk that much, but it was so nice to be out there together!!!

"We headed up to Kris's family's house for Father's Day. We had so many birthdays, graduations and fathers to celebrate. I stuck to my plan and actually did pretty well. I spent most of the time enjoying the company of my adult nieces and nephews."

This might be a highlight of Suzanne's whole journey—a walk with her husband, at his suggestion. Sometimes people think money will make them happy. Suzanne will be the first to tell you Kris's gesture meant more to her than any material thing he could have bought her.

Thursday, June 21

I arrived at the park at 7:30 a.m. and it was a gorgeous 66-degree day with a slight breeze. To throw her off again, I parked down by the tennis courts. We hugged hello then Suzanne said, "Does it get any better than this?"

We spread out a mat in the grass and went over some exercises. While doing a biceps curl, her muscles were showing. Suzanne said that recently she had flexed her muscles for someone. This is a positive sign.

A guy was cutting the grass while we were working out and he was definitely hanging around our area. "He's got the whole stinking park."

We talked about the daily exercises. "You've made that so it's like brushing my teeth." She talked about taking out her contacts, doing some exercises, brushing her teeth, doing some exercises and so on.

"We've never talked about diet pills or diet drinks and you know my love of food." I explained that I don't believe in pills or meal replacement shakes because that won't teach her how to eat. Suzanne still loves food, which means she needs to learn to eat anything she wants…in moderation.

As we walked to my car she said, "I'm getting nervous!" I showed her the lacrosse sticks and balls. "Oh, my gosh, that's gonna be scary! You do remember I got cut from the lacrosse team?"

We threw the ball to each other for a while, then Suzanne said, "I know what's coming up next," and moved the stick into her left hand. At the rate we were going throwing right-handed, it would be too dangerous to play lacrosse left-handed. We ran up and down the field throwing to each other and did more running because of missing the ball. "We have lacrosse sticks somewhere." Great! Now Suzanne can play lacrosse with her sons.

We walked back to the car and I pulled out a basketball. "Oh, my gosh!" Suzanne dribbled the ball down the road to the basketball court. She made shots and ran after the ball when she missed shots. I had her do some full-court running and shooting. On her last run, "I think I peed myself! It's from having children."

After ten minutes she was winded and announced, "I'm out of shape. No, I'm not going to say that!" I could hear her breathing but it subsided quickly, which is a good sign. As we walked back to the car, she dribbled the ball left-handed, her weaker side.

"Ian got a basketball for his birthday." She has yet another sport to play with her children. Suzanne said she could bike to the park with the kids and would put the equipment in a knap sack. Great idea!

Suzanne shared a story about Ian getting better at swimming. "You could see the confidence on his face!" She knows that feeling.

We hugged goodbye then off she went to pick up the boys and take them to swim practice.

Suzanne's Journal Notes …

"I met with Linda in the park for another surprise workout. I really, really enjoy the playing part of exercise. I now need to try and schedule more of that time with the boys!"

An entry like that is priceless!

Friday, June 22

Suzanne's Journal Notes …

"7:00 a.m., 30-minute jog through the park and back. The weather does not get any better than today! Now I am trying to stick to my morning schedule that I set up for myself, and so far I like it. I have checked messages at the office (none!), checked work e-mail and personal e-mail, updated my journal and now I am about to do a few minutes of paperwork before I get my shower."

For Suzanne, jogging isn't a chore, it's something she enjoys doing. She schedules it into her day so it gets done.

Saturday, June 23

Suzanne's Journal Notes ...

"I woke up quite hungry this morning, so I decided to weigh myself—138—not bad for a Saturday. I stayed in bed kind of late this morning and finished my book. It was fiction, but inspired by a family in the Western Virginia Mountains. It was set in 1940. I really enjoyed the book and it made me want to learn more about my ancestors and their struggles and how they lived.

"I decided that it was time to get the garden going that I have been prepping for over a month. I killed all the grass and weeds along the deck in order to start a three-foot garden border down the front of the deck. I purchased all the plants today in hopes that I can get them planted tomorrow. Other than lugging the plants around, I had no real exercise today. Kris and I were going to go for a walk, but it just didn't work out.

"Dinner: 7:00 p.m., we had friends over. We had cheese and crackers with grapes and strawberries, yummy steak on the grill, I made fresh pesto and pasta and Carol brought a delicious salad and bread. I made cupcakes for dessert (but I only had one bite of Kris'). I had two wine & tonic drinks and water. It was a great night to be out on the deck. The kids all enjoyed a game of hide & seek out in the dark, and it was also nice to get to talk with their kids."

Suzanne and Kris are a very social couple; they either go out or have people over. She's able to lose weight because she watches what she eats. There's been a noticeable change in her appetizers; they're more healthful.

Sunday, June 24

Suzanne's Journal Notes ...

"We all worked outside together to get the plants planted. Even though I wasn't doing formal exercise, I think I got a lot of exercise digging the holes, planting the plants and spreading the dirt/mulch. Even if it wasn't exercise, my body felt like it was! I was also drinking tons of water. Later we all went to the movies together. We haven't been to the movies with all five of us in a long time. The movie was great! 10:00 p.m., daily routine."

Working outside definitely counts as exercise; it's cross-training. Suzanne could have opted not to exercise at night but she did.

Tuesday, June 26

Suzanne's Journal Notes ...

"I found out while sitting on the sidelines at KJ's game that the Brazilian delegates are arriving Thursday morning at 10:15 a.m.—an entire day earlier than everyone else, and lucky me, I have to rearrange my entire schedule to accommodate them. I was so mad when I found out. I know that part of the reason I was so mad is because I am stepping out of my comfort zone to host these kids. I have no idea who they are, what they like to eat, how much English they will speak, etc., etc. And I also had a meeting with Linda and lunch with Linda and Bronwyn, who has been on the calendar for a long time that I will have to reschedule. And...the house is certainly not ready yet."

Wednesday, June 27

I received an email with "Scheduling problem!" in the subject line:

"Good Morning Linda. The short story is that I am going to have to cancel both of our meetings tomorrow. I can't tell

you how mad I am! The situation is that we agreed to host this weekend, two 14-year-old boys from Brazil who are coming here to be part of a three-week camp. All the kids who are coming to the camp stay with a host family for the weekend while the chaperones set up the camp. All the delegates are supposed to be arriving on Friday. Well, I found out last night that our delegates are arriving at 10:15 a.m. on THURSDAY! Needless to say I have lost an entire day of preparing for these boys and I had the entire day planned!!! I know we had to wait a long time to get a time to meet Bronwyn for lunch, so I am hoping we will still be able to reschedule.

"You know me well enough that you know I don't like MY schedule messed up—not to mention that this whole hosting thing takes me out of my comfort zone. I know it will all be fine, but I can't believe that they couldn't tell us the flight information less than two days before they were scheduled to arrive. Anyway, now I have to get busy washing sheets and cleaning bedrooms!"

Suzanne does like to be prepared for things and takes so much pride in her home. And she is not one to cancel appointments.

Suzanne's Journal Notes ...

"Lunch: 1:00 p.m., leftover flank steak and the last little bit of the potato salad and not quite the last of the couscous salad. It's a good thing that that salad keeps well. I had a seltzer and a cupcake. It took me until about now to get over being so mad about the Brazil situation. I finally decided to just chill out about it and concentrate on the positive experience this should be for all of us. They are kids and they shouldn't be too concerned about how clean the house is. As long as their beds are clean and we have food in the house, it should work out fine.

"We had to be at the YMCA at 4:15 p.m. for the boys' first swim meet. This was our first official swim meet and I had no idea how long it would be. We were at the meet until 9:00 p.m. They had a small snack bar set up, so I had half of a soft pretzel, 24 ounces of water and a handful of pretzel nuggets. It was so long!! I can't remember the last time I was in one place that long.

"Dinner: 9:30 p.m., we did the fast food drive-thru and I had a grilled chicken sandwich—no fries—and water. I blew it tonight and didn't do my daily routine."

Suzanne hasn't had fast food in quite awhile. She ordered a healthful meal—grilled chicken sandwich with no fries. And the amount of times she's missed doing her daily exercise routine can be counted on one hand. These things contribute to her success.

Thursday, June 28

Suzanne's Journal Notes ...

"10:10 a.m., I arrive at the airport. I knew the flight from Brazil to NYC was on time, but when I got to the airport, I found out that their flight from NYC was delayed, and delayed and delayed—they finally arrived at 2:15 p.m. I had a low-fat carrot muffin and a mango smoothie at the airport—no other choices other than the coffee shop. Oh—and my short-term parking turned long-term and cost me $38! Now I must say, now that I have picked up the kids, I have relaxed greatly. They seem great. They arrived very hungry and you'd think tired, but they have been playing since they got to our house.

"4:00 p.m., I had a veggie burger, a few nacho chips and fruit, 10 ounces of water.

"Dinner: 8:30 p.m., the boys all decided on pizza for after KJ's soccer game, which Kiko got to play in. I had one slice of plain pizza and 24 ounces of water.

"10:00 p.m., another 24 ounces of water and the daily routine."

Suzanne got right back on track and did her daily exercise routine.

Friday, June 29

Suzanne's Journal Notes ...

"6:30 a.m., 30-minute jog through the park. I am so slow that both of the other ladies out there jogging passed me like I was standing still. I did manage to do a couple of intervals in there and I did get a little bit further up Taylor Avenue before I hit the 30-minute mark."

Saturday, June 30

Suzanne's Journal Notes ...

"We got all the boys up early today for our 10:00 a.m. appointment to do the Duck Tour in Philadelphia.

"Lunch: 12:00 p.m., since we were in Philadelphia with Kiko and Gabriel, we thought it would be fun to go to Pat's Steaks. I had a cheese steak with mushrooms, peppers and onions. Boy was that good. I only ate a couple of fries and had a diet soda. That was a real treat. The Duck Tour was fabulous. I would recommend it to anyone. Having lived in this area my entire life, I still got so much out of it. It was fun for the kids because it wasn't too long (about an hour), and the tour guide was really funny and told us all kinds of interesting facts. It really made me want to stay in the city and do more touristy stuff, but I was over-ruled by all the men!

"Dinner: 6:00 p.m., all the host families and their delegates were invited to a picnic. It was really fun to watch these kids from eight different countries (Germany still hasn't arrived) interact and meet each other. I think they are going to have a great camp experience. The boys already picked out the hot chicks in the group, too! I had a turkey burger (no cheese) that I put my salad on top of and coleslaw on top of that. It was really good. I had two pieces of potato salad and fruit. I had 32 ounces of water, but my downfall was dessert. I had two cookies, a piece of pound cake and a big bite of some chocolate dessert. The pound cake was already sliced, and I should have just cut it in half (or less), but I didn't."

Instead of avoiding the desserts and depriving herself, Suzanne was able to eat the desserts she wanted.

In June Suzanne faced the challenge of the boys being out of school and the number on the scale increasing. The latter is a tough one but we found out why. She was reintroduced to baseball, soccer, lacrosse and basketball, all sports she can play with her sons. She came up with games and actually participated in them at Ian's school picnic. A highlight of the month was a walk with her husband Kris, his suggestion. Additional reasons for her success include having a routine and planning.

To Do:

1. Adjust your schedule to accommodate summer months

2. Plan what you're going to do

3. No matter what happens, continue to schedule exercise into your day

4. If you're using a scale as your guide, confirm that it is set to zero each time you use it

July:
Our Last Meeting

Sunday, July 1

Suzanne's Journal Notes ...

"7:30 a.m., 30-minute jog to and through the park.

"Dinner: 6:00 p.m., we took the boys visiting with us to Wabi Sabi for dinner. They had both said that Japanese was their favorite kind of food, so we treated all of us. I think they had fun. It was great to watch how the conversation and especially the laughter picked up as the weekend went on. I had five pieces of sushi for appetizer and steak and shrimp for dinner. I had one Light Kirin beer and 16 ounces of water. We stopped at Rita's for water ice after dinner, but I didn't have anything."

Suzanne is enjoying her company, the boys from South America, with less of an emphasis on the food. And she is listening to her body; she was full so she didn't have water ice.

Tuesday, July 3

I was already at the studio when Suzanne came in with her step. She gave me a big hug and wow—she looked good! The last time we saw each other her weight was 140 and now she's 138. She was hoping for 137 this morning, which would have been a 20-pound weight loss.

Suzanne and Kris went to the mall last evening and she tried on size 6 shorts, which fit. The last time she could fit in that size was about 20 years ago. Prior to our meeting, her sizes were 10s and 12s. She has only one pair of shorts that fit her now; the rest are too big. What will she do with her size 10s and 12s? "I don't know. They're taking up space." She had a pair of pants altered and Kris said they were still too baggy. She said, "People have their fat and skinny clothes, but I'm not doing that." Last year she had purchased size 12 shorts and they "fell off" when she recently tried them on.

We talked about taking pictures in her old clothes so we can see then versus now. If she wanted, she could take one final bike pants and sports bra photo.

"I was really, really hoping for 137 this morning." Losing 19 pounds is amazing for someone who initially didn't have weight loss as a goal.

I told Suzanne she had exceeded my expectations and with a glow on her face she said, "Really?" Yes, I knew she'd lose some weight, but I am excited that she lost 19 pounds. I told her that her dedication to working out and keeping the journal were impressive. Some clients can't keep a journal or exercise for more than a few days and she said, "Why? They're paying you to help them." There are many reasons why, but clients who make our working together a priority are the ones who succeed. "I'm good at following directions." This is another personality trait that made Suzanne successful.

We started doing some exercises with rubber bands when Suzanne said, "Are these new bands? I can't even move them." They were. Rubber bands or certain exercise equipment lose elasticity over time and need to be replaced. Something else was new—her muscles.

Suzanne told me she stepped for 30 minutes yesterday. I haven't asked her to increase her time; she's doing it on her own. Fast Feet are not in her current routine but to challenge herself Suzanne said, "I'm still doing them!"

"This is step routine number five, wow!" We went through the moves and there is definitely an athlete in her body waiting to come out. During the Fast Feet I could hear her breathing, but nothing like when we first did them. It amazed me how quickly she caught on to the moves and patterns and didn't have to rely on her notes.

This routine took about six minutes and thirty seconds. "So this routine is not done?" Nope! Again, Suzanne picked it up almost immediately. She's quite the stepper and will now be able to mix and match all the different step routines.

Suzanne and her family are going away for the Fourth of July holiday, so she'll take the exercise band and strap with her. Months ago Suzanne didn't understand why her friends took their workout gear on their vacation in Philadelphia. Now, she is planning what she's going to take and what she's going to do on vacation—hike in the mountains.

"Hate to exercise and run," she said with her step in her hand. I got a sweaty hug and off she went.

As I was driving to my next appointment I was sad—really sad, because I'll miss Suzanne. She holds a special place in my heart. She has been an awesome client and has done so much more than I imagined. She did an incredible amount on her own and took the initiative to do even more. I wasn't there. I don't live with her. It was all her. I saw Suzanne one day a week, but she knew I was there every day in spirit and just a phone call or email away. I know she enjoyed her journey and I was thankful to be a part of it. Now she is on her own. She has gained control of her life and isn't floundering anymore. Suzanne has created such healthy habits along the way. She will continue with her daily routines, cardio workouts, new sports, playing with her sons, working out with her fitness friends (she's one of them now), watching what she eats, journaling and most importantly, enjoying life. Her life is different and it should be. She's much more confident. She's in control. She walks differently. She even talks differently. It's all good and many more good things will be coming her way! Suzanne is an inspiration to others.

Wednesday, July 11

Suzanne was in the audience of my "Finding Time to Work Out" presentation, so I shared some of her story with the group. Afterward she told someone about her running story: cut from the lacrosse team 30 years ago, felt it was because she couldn't run, didn't run for 30 years, set her May goal to run a half-mile, ran it with me by her side, got emotional during the run, then pumped her fists in the air like "Rocky" (the movie about the boxer) when she finished running 20 minutes. It looked like Suzanne had tears in her eyes as she was telling the story. I had goose bumps.

After her story, the ultimate thing happened—someone asked Suzanne to run with her next year in a 5K race. Almost without hesitation Suzanne agreed to do it. "Linda's suggested it and I feel I can run." No matter what is on my calendar in May of next year, I will be at Suzanne's 5K with camera in hand, taking photos of her race. Actually, I think Suzanne might run a race sooner but I haven't said anything to her about it—it has to be her decision to do it and to have the courage to say yes. I wonder if her fitness friends might encourage her to run a race between now and next May. Maybe Suzanne will encourage her fitness friends to enter a race! The possibilities are endless.

Suzanne has been an absolute joy to work with and I'll miss her terribly. But, she's ready to go on to bigger and better things. I might be called in for a tune-up or maybe a new routine or possibly help train her for something new. Whatever she needs, I'm here for her.

With a lump in my throat and misty eyes, I say goodbye to Suzanne. She has a strong mind and strong body so she can do this on her own. Suzanne is going to be fine and I know in my heart that more good things are coming her way.

Suzanne, have fun with your new life. You look amazing!

TO DO:

1. Reassess what you've done over the last six months

2. Make these next six months even better

Epilogue
by Suzanne Jackson

Linda and I met weekly for just over six months; however, those meetings were just the beginning of my journey and since our last meeting I have had many additional positive life-changing events, lessons, etc.

I continued to jog and even packed my sneakers on our annual vacation to the Outer Banks, shortly after my last session with Linda. I ran five out of the seven days of our vacation! We had been going to the same spot in the Outer Banks for at least four years and I never had known that the community had a fitness center; last year I discovered it on one of my runs. In fact, I saw much more of the area because I spent the time running or walking around.

On our vacation, I bought a new bikini top and decided to wear my bikini on the beach in front of everyone. I wasn't sure about wearing it in front of my family—it made me more nervous than wearing it in front of strangers in Puerto Rico—but I even wore it to play football with my son KJ and his friend Collin!

In August, just two months after my weekly meetings with Linda ended, my friend Caitlin emailed me about running in the Boy Scout 5K race. I had been watching the event for years. Every year the runners start from the park and run right past our house. I always stand out on the driveway and cheer for friends and acquaintances as they run. I remember feeling jealous that they could participate in a 5K and it was inspirational to see young children running with their parents in the race. It's not a race about winning; it is a race about participation. When Caitlin asked me to run I thought she was crazy, but only for a moment. After I thought about it, I knew that if I didn't try it then, I never would. I decided to go for it.

The weekend before the race I decided to practice running the distance of a 5K race. I didn't actually measure out how far I ran, but I ran to the park and went around both loops and home again. It was hard, but I kept going. As I was running up the last leg to our house, I got very emotional again when I realized that I had what it takes to do a 5K. I had run the distance I set out to run, without stopping.

I managed to talk KJ and Griffin into doing the 5K with me. I knew that KJ would run much faster than I because he was in great shape from soccer, but I thought that maybe Griffin would run with me at my pace. On the day of the race I wasn't nervous; I knew I could finish the run because I had done it the week before. KJ took off way in front of me with our neighbor who runs all the time. Griffin decided to run with his best friend, so once again I was on my own. I was slow but steady. As I got to our house, Kris and Ian were cheering me on from the driveway. That was great! As I passed the 2-mile mark, I turned onto a new street and there was Griffin. He was sort of walking and waiting for me at the same time. We continued on together. We were running with some of his other friends from school and Griffin started to hang back with them, but as we got to the home stretch I yelled back that I expected him to finish with me. As we entered the park, and the finish line, Griffin took hold of my hand and said, "We've got this mom. I know you can do it. Let's finish the race." So Griffin and I finished the race, hand in hand, through the finish line. I made it in just under 40 minutes. I think the winner did the race in about 16 minutes. As Griffin and I ran for the finish line, there was KJ, standing on the sideline cheering us on. Linda, Mom, Caitlin and other friends who had already finished were also cheering us on to the finish. It was so great to have such support. Linda knew how much that race meant to me, and I will never forget her being there for me. She took many pictures so the memory will always stay fresh in my mind.

I did another 5K that November and managed to shave about four minutes off my time. To this day I still can't believe I can run!

That September Kris and I started ballroom dance classes through the local adult night school. We both have always loved to dance, so this seemed like the perfect opportunity to get out and move together. It turned out to be so much fun. We spent the whole time giggling and it felt like we were on a date each week.

Kris and I went on a vacation to Italy in October. In preparation for our trip I needed to go through my clothes; I was going to wear some of my pants that I hadn't worn since the previous season. It was amazing to me how big they were. I took six pairs of pants in to be altered. I even had to take back the two pairs of pants that I had bought in February so they could be taken in. When I bought those pants in February, I thought they were my "skinny" pants. It felt so good to have to get all those pants taken in. I also pulled clothes out of my closet that I hadn't worn in years.

When Linda and I first met, I did not set a weight goal. At that time I didn't have the confidence that I could achieve a weight goal; I only knew I wanted to feel better about myself. But if I had said a weight goal out loud, it would have been to weigh 135 pounds by the time we left for our trip to Italy in October. On the morning we left the scale read 134.6 pounds. I felt I had really accomplished a dream come true. Our trip to Italy was awesome. I know the trip was made better by how much better I felt about myself. I didn't obsess about how much I ate, but I was conscious of when to stop eating.

Food has always been such a priority for me. In October the Boy Scouts were selling popcorn. In previous years, I would have ordered only my favorite, but this year I let the kids pick out what they wanted with no regard for what I would have preferred. That way, I wouldn't eat it all! It may sound simple, but I am so in love with food, I have never bought, ordered or cooked anything that I didn't like.

I went out for dinner to a really nice restaurant with my friend Laura. Laura is an avid exerciser and she is tiny. We had a lot to talk about because there is so much going on in both of our lives. I ordered the soup, our favorite appetizer and we shared a dessert. I am definitely not known for skipping the entrée, but even though we were in a wonderful restaurant, we didn't need to go overboard with the food. The evening was about catching up with each other.

Kris called one afternoon and asked me if I was sitting down. He had been offered a temporary assignment in the UK and asked if I would consider it. Of course I would! I have spent almost my entire life living in the same township. Our kids go to my old schools. We still go to the same church that I have been attending since I was 10 years old. If Kris had been given this opportunity at this time last year I think I would have curled up into a ball and hidden in the corner. But now I feel much more confident about life's possibilities and the opportunity to go to the UK sounded like a wonderful adventure for our family. This has been quite a change in my attitude.

Linda advised me that you have to get through a year of experiences in order to get through the holidays, celebrations, vacations, etc. to see how you are going to do and what choices you are going to make. She also advises her clients to maintain and not gain during the holidays. I had set a goal to be not over 140 pounds after the holidays. On January 1, after eating a very late dinner and having dessert and wine, I chose not to put off getting on the scale. After all, it was my day to weigh in and it was the first day of the year. I weighed 140 pounds. Three days later I was back down to 138.

It has been over a year, but the learning and experiences continue. Linda asked me back in the fall if I would speak with Kasey, a personal trainer who works with Linda, at a meeting of a women's organization. At first I didn't feel qualified to speak with any authority, but after we discussed my role, I happily signed on to tell my story. It was a reflective time as I organized what I wanted to share with the group. Organizing my experience on paper also motivated me to keep it up and it helped me to see how far I had come.

The women with whom I was honored to share my story were so lovely. I felt very comfortable working with Kasey and I think they all enjoyed our discussion.

Along came February, when I chose to stop keeping up with my daily journal. It was tax season again and I felt confident that I would stay on track and I continued to weigh myself every Tuesday and Friday morning. I had made the commitment to myself to keep the journal for a year and I achieved that goal. I had been consistent with the exercise routine, so I wasn't worried about slacking off.

Kris and I celebrated our 20th wedding anniversary in May during a long weekend in Puerto Rico. Kris had to be there for a meeting, so it offered a great opportunity for us to celebrate our anniversary. Once again I packed my sneakers and workout clothes. We were in a different hotel, so I did my research before we left to check on the hotel's workout facilities. This time, instead of just admiring the people who were running on the treadmills, I became one of the people running on the treadmills. I was quite nervous to try the treadmill but I got over my nerves and went for it. I can't say that I loved it, but it got the job done. I also wore my bikini the entire time we were poolside.

In June I realized that I hadn't journaled for four months and my weight had gone up a couple of pounds. I decided that I needed to write down my weight and exercise. I need the accountability. I am not writing down all the details of everything I am eating every day, but I am trying to capture as much as I can. My weight went to just above 140, consistently, and I don't like it. I figure that getting back to journaling is my first line of defense.

In July Linda told me she wanted to get together with me and show me a new piece of equipment. We met and she introduced me to Gliding Discs. They look like Frisbees without the lip around the edge. How hard could they be and what could we possibly do with them? I soon discovered that I had myself stuck in a rut of doing the same arm and abs routines at night and that there is a whole world of challenging exercises still waiting for me out there. The exercises were more challenging than any of the other routines Linda had shared with me last year. Even though I was still doing my "daily routine," I had become complacent with the exercises and was not pushing myself to the next level. It was a perfectly timed wake-up call as I was struggling to take off the couple of extra pounds I had put on.

We took our annual trip to the Outer Banks again. My attitude about exercise was different from last year. Last year I felt like I had to prove it to myself that I could exercise during our family vacation. I was so happy that I had run five of the seven days and had discovered so much more of the area where we stayed. This year I approached the vacation exercise knowing that I would join the community gym for the week and felt confident that the exercise would fit naturally into the pace of my vacation. I didn't have the same sense of urgency that I had had the year before. I had four terrific workouts at the gym and it felt like it belonged as part of my vacation. I even had the pleasure of my niece Cassidy's company for two of my workouts. Cassidy is 14 and very active on her travel soccer team. As part of her conditioning for soccer, she participates in a training program. It was so fun for us to share some of our exercises with each other. She led me through some of her abs and weights routines and I did the same with her. It was really neat to have the workout time to share with her. We jogged over to the gym together and did our respective cardio routines, followed by the weights and abs and a walk back to our house.

I also discovered another something new this year, simply because I was working out. From my vantage point on the cardio machine, I could see something in the lake outside. After my workout I decided to walk out and figure out what I was seeing. As I walked out a father and his four kids also were walking toward the lake with a bag of bread. What I discovered was a lake full of turtles. I was able to share my find with the rest of my family and we took two walks to feed the turtles after dinner.

One day while on vacation, after I got back from the gym my mom asked me why I was going to the gym. I think she meant going to the gym rather than just walking the beach for exercise. I paused for a moment to collect my thoughts and realized that I had joined the gym simply because I could join the gym for the week. It was an entire week of vacation with no particular time schedule. At home we spend so much time on a schedule and I figure that on vacation I have time, so I can work out. I know that in the gym I can measure the workout in time, calories, distance, sweat, etc. and get it done. I certainly enjoyed walking on the beach, but that was my bonus exercise; I didn't need to think about how hard I was working out.

I came home from this year's vacation feeling relaxed, successful and motivated to pick up the pace of my workouts, get rid of those couple of extra pounds and enjoy the habits that I have developed over the last 19 months.

When I started my fitness journey I was size 10/12 and now I'm size 6/8. I do the cardio workout at least four times and sometimes five times per week. I do the step routine, run or bike. On top of that, I spend many evenings walking with the kids and Tucker. I wouldn't call it a cardio workout, but it has been great being outside and taking advantage of the time with the family. The daily routine includes legs on the Gliding Discs or with the strap, arms with weights or the strap and abs with the Gliding Disc, the strap or with no equipment. I usually do five different arm exercises, five different abs exercises and 20 push-ups each time.

Exercise has become a habit in my life. I can feel it in my body when I need to work harder. I have spent more time in exercise-type activities with the kids, even if it is just a walk after dinner. I feel I have more control over my life, although there still are times when I feel completely overwhelmed and need to take a time-out to get my head back in the game. I feel so much better in my clothes and it is much more fun shopping for clothes.

Without a doubt, I will keep exercise in my life. I know I have plenty of choices when it comes to exercise and I can see changing it up with different types of activities. I don't want to be locked into one form of exercise, but I am completely educated on how to avoid this problem. I would like to potentially add an exercise class or a dance class to my weekly routine. My biggest difficulty is paying attention to my food portions; I can easily get into trouble when I stop focusing on how much I am eating.

One year after my first Boy Scout 5K race, I ran it again. No fanfare this time, just plenty of mental games with myself. I ran it in 38:09. It was a beautiful day and my neighbors were there and we all cheered each other on. I am so glad I did it!!!

What else has changed in my life? I recently got a new job with a 50% pay increase. I finally had the confidence to ask for what I feel I am really worth! On a family note, we joined the local YMCA and I took my first fitness class in eight years!

My journey started with the intent of getting my body to be healthier— I never imagined just how healthy my whole life would become!